Arlena Siobhan Liggins
Making Diabetes

Medical Humanities | Volume 2

This book is dedicated to the wonderful and brave people in Uganda, who have shared such intimate parts of their lives with me.

Arlena Siobhan Liggins completed her doctorate in Anthropology at the University of Bayreuth in 2018. She works as a Scientific Officer at the DLR Project Management Agency within the field of Global Health.

Arlena Siobhan Liggins
Making Diabetes
The Politics of Diabetes Diagnostics in Uganda

[transcript]

Zugl.: Bayreuth, Univ., BIGSAS, Diss., 2018.

Published with the support of the Bayreuth International Graduate School of African Studies (BIGSAS)

Bibliographic information published by the Deutsche Nationalbibliothek
The Deutsche Nationalbibliothek lists this publication in the Deutsche Nationalbibliografie; detailed bibliographic data are available in the Internet at http://dnb.d-nb.de

© 2020 transcript Verlag, Bielefeld

All rights reserved. No part of this book may be reprinted or reproduced or utilized in any form or by any electronic, mechanical, or other means, now known or hereafter invented, including photocopying and recording, or in any information storage or retrieval system, without permission in writing from the publisher.

Cover layout: Maria Arndt, Bielefeld
Cover picture: Arlena Siobhan Liggins

Print-ISBN 978-3-8376-4897-3
PDF-ISBN 978-3-8394-4897-7
https://doi.org/10.14361/9783839448977

Contents

Abbreviations 7

Introduction 9
Traveling tools, traveling methods 14
The matter with numbers 17
Spaces of diabetes – the fieldsites 21
Sketching Uganda's health care system 23
A roadmap to visibility – outline of the book 26

1. "If you are lacking insulin" – Diabetes Mellitus 29
Not just about sugar 30
The mysterious illness: one (hi)story of diabetes 34
A disease without (hi)story? 39
From urine to blood 41
Testing matters: diagnostic tests and diagnostic criteria 44

2. (Un)measured yet (un)seen 51
Number business 55
Data in transit? A status quo of NCDs in Uganda 61
(Un)measured but seen – diabetes in Uganda 66

3. Thinking beyond the evident 73
Technologies without borders? 73
The rise of evidence-based medicine 77
Infrastructures or "Stuff, staff, space and systems" 84
Translation(s) in a technologized world 89

4. A 'simple' technology and its translations: the glucometer 97
Know it, get it started and "make your life easier" 101
Not for diagnosis? 108
Keeping the testing going 115

5. Diagnostic detours and a logic of chance ... 119
Diagnostic (un)certainties ... 124
Private Diagnostics ... 129
Survival of the richest ... 133
Pending diagnoses and "technological flowers" ... 137
Diagnosis as a logic of chance? ... 141

6. My numbers and my-Self ... 149
"Numbers don't lie" ... 155
Knowing the good number ... 160
"Who shall I trust more, the number or myself?" ... 166
Numbers against uncertainty, numbers for a hopeful life ... 171

7. Seek and you shall find: Medical Outreaches ... 177
The crowd pullers ... 184
"An act of giving without receiving" ... 189
"The money is totally worth the experience" ... 196
Desired tests, undesired outcomes? ... 203

Concluding Remarks ... 209
Contesting the global health agenda ... 210
Trajectories of a fluid technology ... 211
Re-visiting (in)visibility ... 214

References ... 217

Abbreviations

ADA American Diabetes Association

AIDS Acquired Immune Deficiency Syndrome

ART Antiretroviral Therapy

BP Blood Pressure

DAH Development Assistance for Health

DFG Deutsche Forschungsgemeinschaft

DHO District Health Officer

DKA Diabetic ketoacidosis

DM Diabetes Mellitus

EBM Evidence-based medicine

HC Health Center

HIV Human Immuno-Deficiency Virus

HLM High-level meeting

HMIS Health Management Information System

IDF International Diabetes Federation

IHME Institute for Health Metrics and Evaluation

JMS Joint Medical Stores

LMIC Low- and middle-income country

MDG Millennium Development Goal

MoH Ministry of Health

MRC Medical Research Council

NCD Non-communicable disease

NDA National Drug Authority

NMS National Medical Stores

NTD Neglected tropical disease

OGTT Oral Glucose Tolerance Test

PEPFAR The U.S. President's Emergency Plan for AIDS Relief

RCT Randomized Control Trial

SDG Sustainable Development Goal

STC Socially transmitted condition

STS Science and Technology Studies

UDHS Uganda Demographic and Health Survey

UGX Uganda Shilling

UICC Union internationale contre le cancer

UN United Nations

UNICEF United Nations International Children's Emergency Fund

USD US Dollars

VHT Village Health Team

WDF World Diabetes Federation

WHO World Health Organization

Introduction

It happened on June 5th in the year 2009[1]. A Friday, 26 degrees Celsius. The wind was blowing lightly and the average humidity measured that day was 78%. A thunderstorm would be looming over Kampala, the capital city of Uganda, later in the day. It was also that very day in June, when a 42-year old man, whom I will name George, died only a few hours after he had been seen by a medical doctor. The newspaper article in the Daily Monitor, one of the two biggest national newspapers in Uganda, reports that George was a painter living with his mother. Only one week before he died, George started to become restless and began drinking huge amounts of water. He and his mother were thinking that it was likely that he had developed a heat stroke, which would surely pass. However, instead of improving, George's condition worsened and culminated in a state of confusion, lethargy and stupor and "his speech was incoherent". His mother discerned that her "son's breathing was erratic and his eyes were sunken and his breath had a queer smell". One day before his death, on June 4th at 5.50 p.m., so the article says, George's mother consulted a health care worker who knew about George's history of depression. She sent for a doctor because his condition was worrying. George's mother would later tell the court that "the doctor did not have any equipment on him" when he attended to George. The doctor's diagnosis: depression. He gave the advice to visit his general practitioner the following day in order to receive medication. The last time his mother saw her son alive was at 1a.m. Five hours later, when she wanted to check on him again, her son "had died in bed". After George's death had been investigated by the police, the case finally ended up in court. One of the expert witnesses, a medical professor, explained that he had concluded that all of George's symptoms, the "state of confusion, thirst, sunken eyes, peculiar breath,

---

1 This narration is freely told following the newspaper article "Wrong diagnosis lands doctor in jail" published in the Daily Monitor on December 11th 2016, by Dr. Sylvester Onzivua. The quotes in the narration are taken from this article. The emphases in the quotes are mine. The original article can be found here: http://www.monitor.co.ug/artsculture/Reviews/Wrong--diagnosis--doctor-jail/691232-3480400-wtljvbz/index.html.

and inability to speak [were] classic symptoms of diabetic keto-acidosis[2]". He continued that it would have been the obligation of the doctor to check the sugar levels in the "patient's blood and [he] should have immediately had the patient admitted to hospital where he would have been treated and saved". Another medical expert ascertained the doctor should have measured the blood sugar levels with a glucometer, which would not even have taken one minute. "The *failure to diagnose* the patient's condition was the main cause of death", he concluded. After considering the body of evidence, **the judge pronounced his sentence:** "The nature of your offence is too serious for anything other than a custodial sentence. You failed to *recognise* the patient's condition despite the fact that all the *classic signs* of a diabetic condition were present. You opted for a diagnosis that was *contrary to all the evidence*. This was a gross breach of your duty of care. An expert called your diagnosis appalling. I agree. It was clearly criminally negligent and a wholly preventable death." The doctor who had failed to diagnose George with diabetes was sentenced to two and a half years in prison for manslaughter.

Why did George have to die? Is his medical history of depression to blame, blinding the doctor to consider any other disease as the reason for George's ailments? Or because the doctor who attended to him was not able to interpret and "recognize" the "classic signs" of diabetes? Perhaps the doctor would have been able to diagnose George with diabetes if he had had the equipment to test him, which was seen to be his obligation and "duty of care"? I am afraid these questions will have to remain without clear answers. Conceivably, it is a bit of everything. No matter how much effort we will put in understanding what has really happened to George and especially why it has happened or why it became a legal case in the first place, we do know that the doctor failed to diagnose him with diabetes and instead chose a diagnosis that was "contrary to all the evidence". A diagnostic act hereby appears to be not only critical and essential in clinical practice in the encounter between a patient and a medical practitioner. But a diagnosis is also a political and economic[3] issue, dependent on functioning (health) infrastructures, the availability of and access to tools like diagnostic devices and the knowledge when and how to apply them. I shall utilize George's story to mark the course this book will pursue.

This book examines diagnostic and testing practices in the case of diabetes in Uganda. What seems to be the story of a single individual, 42-year old George, can in fact be seen as part of a larger problem: Matters of diagnoses especially for diabetes are relevant more than ever in the face of growing numbers of individuals

---

2 Diabetic ketoacidosis (DKA) is an acute life-threatening complication of diabetes (more frequently in type 1 diabetes) characterized by a severe lack of insulin in the bloodstream (cf. Srinivas et al. 2016).
3 And it may become a legal issue as well, as we have seen.

affected with this disease globally. Opposed to the long-held assumption that diabetes is predominantly a concern of countries in the minority world, especially the majority world[4] is now struggling to deal with this chronic disease. Compared to the number of deaths due to HIV/AIDS in 2016, five times as many people died as a consequence of diabetes worldwide – of which three quarters occurred in the majority world (Al-Lawati 2017; Moran-Thomas 2017). In this 21st century, many scholars are warning, a growing "epidemic" of diabetes is dawning (e.g. van Crevel, van de Vijver and Moore 2017; Rodriguez-Fernandez 2016; Herman and Zimmet 2012; Assah and Mbanya 2009; Tabish 2007; Boutayeb 2006; Marshall 2004).

Matters of diagnosis have clearly climbed up on the global health agenda. The appreciation of diagnostics as an integral part of care for the health of the global public has expanded: from a former focus on access to essential medicines in the early years of this millennium, by the question of access to diagnostic tools. As a result, the development of innovative and inexpensive point-of-care devices – allegedly easy to use, mobile devices, applicable even outside of hospital settings – has gained momentum, seeking to enable the rapid detection especially of infectious diseases in resource poor settings (Street et al. 2014 et al.). This is not the case for the glucometer. Compared to humanitarian point-of care devices, specifically designed to meet the needs of under-resourced settings, the glucometer has not been designed to tackle urgent diagnostic issues for places where essential laboratory infrastructures are lacking. As the first and often only choice technology to diagnose diabetes, glucometers, however, take on a significant role in the diagnosis of diabetes particularly in these settings. In a way, glucometers are emblematic for how the access to suitable diagnostic devices for this pressing global health issue is erratically distributed across the globe (Moran-Thomas 2017). While glucometers are seen to be part of the basic health care package in large parts of the minority world, the access to and maintenance of these point-of-care devices may be hard to attain in large parts of the majority world. Yet, since diabetes is a chronic disease, which can be managed but not cured, continuous testing is an essential part of the long-term care needed to determine the amount of medicines in order to keep the glucose levels at bay (Heurtin-Roberts and Becker 1993). Unlike other point-of-care devices the glucometer serves as both, a diagnostic as well as a continuous testing tool. As Moran-Thomas (2017) puts it straight in a recent article, the role of the glucometer "in frontline diagnosis also hinges on a painful irony: glucometers' metrics help to make visible an enormous population of people living with diabetes

---

4 Throughout this book I will avoid using terms such as "Global South", "developing country" or even "third world", unless they are part of a quote. Instead, I prefer the terms "minority world" and "majority world" to focus on the demographic distribution rather than the economic development.

in contexts of poverty, many of whom cannot consistently access the same meters then vital for day-to-day care."

The glucometer is yet part of another predicament. It serves not only as a diagnostic and glucose testing tool, but it is further an epidemiological tool that has a great stake in making diabetes visible and quantifiable in Uganda and beyond. Evidence and the visibility of a disease are interlinked with the diagnostic possibilities, like the story of George has demonstrated and as this book intends to show. Evidence, especially in the form of numbers, is further needed in order to stand up to the regimes of global health. Numbers will be adduced when health priorities are set, when agendas are formulated and action plans for global health interventions are planned and implemented. The equation is simple: the visibility of diabetes stands and falls with the access to appropriate diagnostic technologies. I therefore argue that the restricted availability of glucometers is one reason for why the widely spreading global health claims of dramatically increasing numbers of diabetes are only slowly translated into action on a global scale as well as on a local level in Uganda.

In this regard this book asks: How does the glucometer contribute to the making of diabetes in Uganda and what does the device actually render visible on a local scale and beyond? In seeking to answer this question, a number of other questions emerge. What are the circumstances under which diabetes is diagnosed and tested in Uganda? Which trajectories do individuals with diabetes and their caregivers pursue to access diagnostic devices for diabetes and when do they fail? Who are the actors involved in diagnosing and testing this chronic disease, what are their agendas and how do they deal with the outcomes of these tests? And finally, in which ways does the glucometer help to solve or create new problems in Uganda?

I will approach these questions through the conceptual lenses of evidence-based medicine, infrastructure and translation. Linking these concepts, I suggest, reflects the interwovenness of the technological, infrastructural and scientific apparatus that determines diagnostics and in turn frames care. The global travel of biomedical technologies hereby offers a platform to understand how certain techniques and technologies come to work together in specific infrastructures and under certain premises. Technologies are important constituents of individual and collective practices ordering lives and bodies in health and illness. Therefore, the value of medical technologies and the practices in which they are involved cannot be neglected or simply taken for granted. What happens when a biomedical technology like the glucometer travels to a context distinct from its country of origin (cf. Müller-Rockstroh 2007; Hadolt et al. 2012)?

In 1981 Allan Young made the case for the notion of embedded knowledge, which cannot be deduced from peoples' talks or stories alone but is incorporated in nonverbal schemes, clinical procedures and technologies. Unraveling medical knowledge also requires to look at practices and apparatuses and not only into minds and cognitive operations (Young 1981: 324). In the process of translating and appropriating a technology in a novel context (be it a glucometer or a new policy), neither biomedicine nor its new context stays the same. As they travel and are put to use in diverse environments, biomedical practices and artifacts shape their receiving societies. They do so for example by altering existing practices, bodies, identities, and institutional structures. Simultaneously, the technology itself is formed and created by the cultural, political, economic, and sociocultural dynamisms expressed in these environments. The extent to which biomedical practices and artifacts stay the same or alter in the progression of their appropriation and translation – at home, in clinical settings, global and public health interventions, or in policymaking (Granado et al. 2011) – hence is an empirical matter.

In order to critically employ the legislations of global health (Biehl and Petryna 2013; Adams 2013, 2016), diagnostic and testing practices in the case of diabetes can be a crucial step to get an ample picture of the dynamics within the (re)organization of health care services on a local level, but also the need for a reorganization and reframing of chronic diseases on the global health agenda. Chronic conditions in general and diabetes specifically in Uganda and elsewhere in the majority world can be a crucial entry point to understand how an 'emerging' threat like diabetes is and can be approached and how it is handled. Since diagnostics are not only essential in uncovering disease on an individual level, but contribute to the visibility of diseases in epidemiological terms, I intend to highlight the complexities in which the glucometer is entangled in Uganda. Scrutinizing matters of diagnoses does not only highlight local embroilments, but may allow insights into broader structural and global dynamics that have to be addressed when tackling diabetes as a pressing global health issue. The way diabetes is diagnosed marks what will be made visible and what remains hidden. Therefore, this book ultimately deals with how a biomedical device like the glucometer alongside its consistency and rationalities, contributes to the (in)visibility of diabetes. And this in the light of a setting deprived and curtailed by resource shortages, weak health infrastructures and an alleged lack of global interest and investment.

Up to now, a range of studies on diabetes and other chronic diseases within anthropology and related fields in the social sciences have mainly been conducted in the minority world. For instance, focusing on health beliefs, coping strategies and the day-to-day suffering of individuals affected by diabetes (cf. Lynch and Cohn 2016; Mendenhall 2010; Manderson and Smith-Morris 2010; Guell 2009). Others have highlighted the chronicity, long-term, aspect of this disease (Weaver and Mendenhall 2014; Whyte 2012). I do not question the merit of these studies for they have yielded valuable insights especially for what it means to be chronically ill. The diagnosis of diabetes in weak health infrastructures, however, has not yet been adequately captured. Without attending to the ways in which diagnostic practices are enacted in a setting like Uganda, the daily hazards of dealing with diabetes as a public health issue as well as the struggle for visibility in the vortex of the global diabetes epidemic, will remain unseen.

Accordingly, I see the main contribution of this book in the critical examination of diabetes as an emerging global health problem. The days in which HIV/AIDS, Malaria and Tuberculosis were the major killers in Uganda and elsewhere seem to have passed. Against the odds this shift has not led to a decrease of global interest in these matters but the contrary is the case: the global market for the so-called 'Big Three', HIV/AIDS, tuberculosis and malaria, is flourishing as ever. On the downside, actions taken to tackle diabetes and other chronic diseases do not match the claims of an arising diabetes epidemic. The battle against diabetes surely is an individual and local one, but it is not less a global one. I argue that the faith and hopes towards a technology like the glucometer may obscure the far-reaching implications intrinsic to such a diagnostic device. In the face of the long-term care and continuous testing an individual will need, the glucometer will not be able to serve as a panacea. Instead it raises larger questions about the prioritization of certain health conditions over others. The glucometer hereby is illustrative for the struggle to provide and maintain diagnostic access for diabetes while having to deal with rising numbers of people affected by this disease.

The following section will foreground my research questions on visibilities of diabetes in Uganda in a methodological reflection. I will illustrate the role ethnographic field research may play especially in the evidence-based world we live in today. We will have a closer look at the emergence of the new global health (chapter two) alongside the rise of evidence-based medicine (chapter three) in more detail – ethnographic evidence consistently *"dies* within the dominant conceptual paradigms of global health" (Biehl and Petryna 2013: 16; emphasis in the original).

Traveling tools, traveling methods

> "Put aside the camera, and join […]
> in what is going on" — Malinowski 1984
> [1922]: 20.

This book is based on approximately 14 months of anthropological fieldwork. In 2012, when I came to Uganda for the first time, I conducted three-months of research collecting illness narratives of individuals affected by diabetes for my M.A. dissertation research. Two years later I returned to Uganda as a research assistant for the DFG-funded project "Translating Global Health Technologies: Standardisation and organisational learning in health care provision in Uganda and Rwanda"[5]. The following year, in June 2015, I joined this research project as a PhD candidate, and undertook another nine months of fieldwork in three consecutive research phases[6]. Coming back to Uganda on these different occasions after the initial stay, meant that I had a solid basis on which I could ground my research activities. In a way, it was like continuing from where I had stopped, rather than starting anew when I came back for my official PhD research. Many of the contacts I had established back in 2012 were fruitful also for the current research. For example, I continued my research in two of the three health centers where I spent large parts of my fieldwork. Further, some of the individuals I had worked with before became part of my PhD research again, including diabetes patients and their health care workers.

Semi-structured interviews (Bernard 2011; Medjedovic and Witzel 2010), focus-group discussions (Pérez 2017; Witzel and Reiter 2012), numerous informal conversations and participant observation (Paxson 2017; Robben and Sluka 2007; Lüders 2004) were the main tools that helped me approach my research object and track places and people who were, in one way or the other, involved in making diabetes visible in Uganda. In total I collected 57 formal interviews with diverse actors in the field. These included members of the Ministry of Health of Uganda; employees of the National Medical Store (NMS), responsible for the distribution of medicines and medical equipment in Uganda; I met district health officers as well as biostatisticians; I visited different medical equipment distributers in Kampala; and of course, I worked closely together with laboratory technicians, nurses, doctors and with people affected by diabetes. Next to the formal interviews, a large number of interviews were informal in nature, where I took extensive notes.

I also engaged in participant observations for which I spent a large part of my stay in three governmental health facilities, which I will further specify in the next section. In these settings, I mostly commuted between the examination rooms and the laboratories, following patients and glucometers. I assisted in some of the activities that were going on there. One of my tasks for instance was, to assist in the registration and documentation of the individuals who were seeking care at the governmental health facilities. Especially when a health worker or a laboratory technician was working alone, this meant a small relief for her or him, considering the large amount of paperwork required. At times, there were up to four different books in which the same information had to be written. I noted down patients'

---

5 DFG is the abbreviation for "Deutsche Forschungsgemeinschaft", the organization for science and research in Germany. You can find more details on the research project here: http://www.spp1448.de/projects/translating-global-health-technologies/.
6 The first phase took place between July and September 2015, followed by another phase from January to March 2016. The final research phase was from July to September 2016.

names, their villages, their age and sex. Sometimes I also wrote down the testing results – depending on the health center not only for diabetes, but also for other tests that were performed in the laboratories. I called patients by their names when it was their turn to see the doctor or health care worker, which very often ended up in bouts of laughter, both in the laboratory and the waiting area, since I was apparently not very good at pronouncing the names correctly. At the end of a clinic day I would help to clean the examination room, assist in filling up the shelves with medication. I often gave health workers a ride from the villages back to Kampala. An additional and welcome possibility to ask more questions that had come up during the day, or simply more time to chat about other things.

Though all interviews and focus group discussions were recorded with a digital voice-recorder after obtaining the consent of the interviewee and consequently transcribed verbatim, I took extensive notes. This was also the case if recordings were not possible or unwanted. My field diary was my constant companion fed with information, thoughts, ideas, worries and sketches whenever and wherever possible. This was a welcome routine especially in the evenings after I had returned home and had the time and quiet to reflect upon the day and prepare for the ones to come. Most interviews were conducted in English, however, especially interviews and group discussions with individuals affected by diabetes, even more so in the villages, required the assistance of a translator. Though I had attended a Luganda language class, the language widely spoken in central Uganda, my proficiency remained very limited. Despite my limited vocabulary and grammar, which merely allowed me to engage in simple phrases like saying 'hello' and 'good bye', 'thank you', or 'diabetes', this was nevertheless important to establish a good rapport with people. My informants enjoyed it very much when I tried to speak Luganda and appreciated the effort on my part. My language skills would have not been enough to conduct a whole interview, not to mention grasping the fine nuances and details this language has to offer. I therefore worked very closely with my interpreter Lucy, who is an anthropologist herself. Her support was of indispensable assistance not only during the interviews when translating, but also when debriefing thereafter or arranging the next ones[7].

My aim to study diabetes in terms of its visibility, required me to move around and search where it was made visible, how and by whom. The glucometer is one of the main actors, contributors and facilitators that makes diabetes visible. Since this device is mobile and not fixed or bound to a certain place or actor, it required me to

---

7 At times, I had two interpreters. While Lucy was conducting the interview or leading the focus group, the other interviewer was sitting next to me translating simultaneously. This convenient possibility made it possible for me to ask follow up questions immediately. That I partially had two interpreters was due to the fact that Lucy had a family member whom she was teaching interviewing techniques.

be mobile too. I had to maneuver between different locations, engage with different people and join diverse activities. The empirical chapters of this book (chapter four to seven) reflect this mobility and flexibility, where in each of these chapters different actors engage in (testing) practices for different reasons and with different outcomes. Since the glucometer is a traveling technology this opened up the field to do what Marcus (1995) framed a multi-sited ethnography. As suggested by Marcus (1995) and Hannerz (2003) shadowing a traveling technology and to observe its alterations makes it necessary to study a particular technology or object in different places. Multi-sited ethnography "defines as its objective the study of social phenomena that cannot be accounted for by focusing on a single site […]. The essence of multi-sited research is to follow people and objects, connections, associations, and relationships across space (because they are substantially continuous but spatially non-contiguous)" (Falzon 2009: 1f.). Multi-sited ethnography the way Marcus (1995) suggested, should nevertheless not simply be understood as a proliferation of different sites, stacking one on top of the other. Instead it should rather be perceived as a practice deriving from the object of study, because if "our object is mobile and/or spatially dispersed, being likewise surely becomes a form of participant observation […], it is 'fieldwork as travel practice'" (Falzon 2009: 9). Hence, ethnography itself emerges to a travelling practice following objects like glucometers, other technologies, ideas and people (ibid.).

Depending on the actor, and dependent on the agendas, a certain part of diabetes may become visible or it may remain hidden. Studying the visibility of diabetes in Uganda therefore meant to hunt for the different actors who contributed to it in on one way or the other. Especially in the beginning of the research I caught myself being a 'detective' on the trail of diabetes and the glucometer. I could not take it for granted that I would find one in every health facility. Even if the device was said to be at a certain place, for instance in a specific health facility, this did not necessarily mean that it was (still) there. At the same time, it was possible to find the glucometer in places where I would not have expected it. One time for instance, a glucometer fell out of the pants pocket of a passenger who was sitting next to me in a minibus in Kampala. It could neither be taken for granted that diabetes was captured in numbers in policy documents or at the Ministry of Health of Uganda. Especially in the beginning this made it hard to grasp the scope of this chronic disease until I understood that the fragmented or missing numbers were part of its visibility and invisibility.

The matter with numbers

Diabetes has a lot to do with numbers. From a global health perspective and in line with what evidence-based medicine (see chapter three) tries to reach and convey, disease is inherently bound to numbers. Diabetes is about numbers from an epidemiological point of view, concerning the prevalence rate of the disease in different settings. Individuals become numbers as soon as they are diagnosed with a disease – number 11 in the registration book of a health center, or individual 'number 3789' with diabetes in Uganda.[8] Diabetes itself is expressed through a number, the glucose level that makes a diagnosis possible in the first place, and will be part of the lives of individuals from the day this diagnosis has been declared. Getting a clear picture of these numbers and gathering quantitative data on diabetes, however, appeared to be a difficult undertaking in my research and the information I received varied substantially. The national prevalence rate of 3.3% for diabetes in Uganda had been generated and published in a report from 2016 (MoH 2016; see also chapter two), the first and only study assessing the burden of non-communicable diseases in Uganda. However, it was a lot more difficult to receive localized information on the number of patients having diabetes in the districts, respectively to find what these numbers were based on or how they had been generated. It was further not easy to track down, which health facilities in Uganda were able to diagnose and offer testing and medication for diabetes, for instance as part of functioning diabetes clinic days. On an official level, such as in the Ministry of Health of Uganda, where I expected to find this information, I was looked at with skepticism and suspicion. They wondered, why I would be interested in where or how diabetes was diagnosed or which facility had a diabetes clinic, if the national prevalence rate was finally known? Was it not enough to know *that* diabetes was diagnosed instead of knowing *where* this was? Or, as I was once asked "But what is it more you need to know? The numbers, they are now there." Indeed, numbers, or numerical evidence, are one way to account for the visibility of a disease. But what happens if these numbers are highly localized and in other parts (e.g. other districts of Uganda) fragmented or lacking or not the ones you were seeking for? Or what happens, if numbers cannot express what words can?

Ethnographic methods are often not as valued as data from disciplines that predominantly work with a quantitative methodology and numbers, as is common in many global health studies. Qualitative methods here often have a reputation of not being objective, and therefore not qualified to establish generalizations, which is usually the aim of statistical and numerical evidence that biomedicine and related fields usually operate with. I had sent a chapter of this book to one of my friends, a laboratory technician, working in a laboratory of a governmental health facility in Uganda. A week later he replied in an email that he liked the paper, *but* "I

---

8 There is a registration system partly in place for diabetes in Uganda. Yet it is not, or cannot be used in every health facility across Uganda, which leads to a fragmentation of data in Uganda and a lack of data focused on diabetes in specific areas of Uganda.

think some numbers should be included to make it more meaningful". This statement, adding numbers for more meaningfulness, is not only an expression of the encounter between two individuals with different disciplinary and methodological backgrounds. Instead, rationalizations, numbers and metrics are taken to be the most reliable and trustworthy entities and indicators. They are regarded as the necessary foundations on which (political) actions and considerations about the world can unhesitatingly be grounded. Yet the narratives and stories we come to hear and note down, and which we use to add lived experience are unique ways of dealing with, understanding, and conveying certain phenomena in our ethnographies.

Nevertheless, medical anthropology feeds on biomedical evidence in many ways. As Ecks (2009) highlights, in our funding proposals, or as in my case in the introduction to this book, we use epidemiological data to show that our object of study is urgent in one way or the other. When moving in the realm of the global health today we more than ever before need to ask how medical anthropology is connected to biomedical practice and global health. Ecks (2009) argues that

> the two fields are not as far apart in how they gather evidence as is usually thought. Biomedicine is not a passive object of the anthropological gaze. Instead, biomedicine defines most of the parameters within which we are working. Biomedicine informs anthropology on all levels of inquiry, from the definition of what we aim to study, to the way we write field notes, and the way we stake our claims in arguments with medicine. On each level, questions of 'evidence' are crucial. (ibid.: 82)

Like the story of George in the beginning has shown, there can be evidence and 'visibility' of disease even next to or as a substitute for numbers. It is visibility through stories. As human beings, and perhaps even more so as anthropologists, next to the observations we make and the interviews we conduct, we listen to the (hi)stories of the individuals we come to meet. People with whom we work and share parts of our lives and from whom we want to learn. Each story – the way it is told and what individuals decide to tell – is unique. Stories cannot be captured as a number. While we carefully listen to these (hi)stories and while we spend our days living small parts of these stories with them, new worlds unfold. Hereby, as Mol (2002) states "[m]ethods are not [only] a way of opening a window on the world, but a way of interfering with it. They act, they mediate between an object and its representations" (ibid.: 155). Though numbers count especially in evidence-based medicine, stories like the one of George can enrich these numbers. As Merry (2016) beautifully encapsulates, ethnography is essential

> to counter the homogenization and stripping away of the social world inherent to quantification. Without that, one misses critical dimensions of the texture of social life and reinterprets the loves of the nonelites around the world through

the lens of the cosmopolitan experts who design indicators and their concepts of social problems and interventions [...]. Quantification has a great deal to contribute to global knowledge and governance, but it is important to resist its seductive claim to truth and to recognize it as only one form of knowledge with its own distinctive limitations. The narrative ethnographic account provides an important complement to quantification. We rely on numbers alone at our peril. (ibid.: 221f.)

With stories like George's, we can get noticed, make someone politically aware of a problem, attract the attentiveness of possible donors or "justify sweeping ideas and large-scale interventions" (Biehl and Petryna 2013: 17). Who, if not an anthropologist, is better positioned to capture these stories? It is empirical and not numerical evidence that arises when individuals seek to express their worries or other feelings, their hopes and angers or their happiness. Narratives, "which then open up to complex human stories in time and space. Life stories do not simply begin and end. They are stories of transformation, linking the present to the past and to a possible future" (ibid.: 19).

The way how anthropologists work has changed in a way. It is no longer a stepping in and stepping out the way Hortense Powdermaker insinuated back in 1966. As anthropologists we step in, into novel settings and new situations. When we step out by leaving our 'field', when we go back home, we often times stay connected. We are aware that not only we have changed, but the 'field' has changed, too. Though we might not any longer be present in person, the connected world of today allows us to stay in touch with the individuals we have met and with whom we have built a relationship. We might be thousands of kilometers apart, yet we are always only one message away. "Fieldwork thus emerges as process rather than event, a 'spiralling' cumulative progression which borrows on a number of empirical strands – collaboration, the appointment of field assistants, direct participant observation, Internet research, and so on" (Falzon 2009: 16). Doing fieldwork has a different quality with the technological possibilities there are today. It is a way of working where you can always stay informed by your informants and with this have the possibility of being able to receive and convey information and fill in the gaps retrospectively. The stories we come to hear do not simply end when we leave the 'field', but they may continue through different channels in the future.

I do not want to denigrate fields such as global health that are predominantly concentrating and working with and through numbers. Instead this book will challenge and critically question the premises and highlight some of the consequences a mainly quantitative approach has. We may ponder about whether the methods we use should be put into a hierarchy when it is ultimately the lives of the people we seek to improve. By framing diabetes in terms of its visibility I suggest that numerical evidence might not be that different from ethnographic evidence in terms of making a disease visible. It is the way the results and outcomes are presented that mostly differs. It is then only of secondary relevance to which disciplinary background we belong when we discuss tangible complexities of our lives or when we might render something visible which numbers cannot capture. As anthropologists and social scientists in general, we are not able to change the world for the people we work with, but we can counteract seemingly rigid regimes such as the one of global health by continuing to make the individuals visible and their voices heard by adding life to the impersonality of numbers and statistical evidence.

Spaces of diabetes – the fieldsites

I will briefly introduce the three districts and the main health centers where I spent a large part of my fieldwork and from which most of the empirical material originates. Places, where I met individuals with diabetes, laboratory technicians who diagnosed and tested them, health care workers who attended to the patients and prescribed medicine, and also places where, if available, glucometers assisted them in doing so.

My research was mainly conducted in three governmental health facilities, each located in a different district, which I will call district X, district Y and district Z[9]. In district X and district Y, I had already conducted research on diabetes prior to my PhD studies. Choosing these districts therefore also had pragmatic reasons because I knew the people working there rather well and in turn they knew me and what my research was about and facilitated access. Their proximity to Kampala, where I was based, allowed me to commute back and forth between the different field sites and Kampala. Kampala as the capital was also where the Ministry of Health is located where I interacted closely with officials. Above all I was tied to the availability and possibility of diagnostics for diabetes and therefore it made sense to continue working in these facilities.

Further, these three health facilities (HC) varied from each other in terms of the services they offered for diabetes patients. This diversity proved fruitful especially for comparative reasons: The health center in district X had no separate diabetes clinic; the one in district Z had been in its infant stage of offering a specialized clinic for diabetes; and the health center in district Y had a well attuned diabetes clinic with an experienced diabetes nurse heading it. Overall there are 112 districts in Uganda, divided into different regions, central, eastern, northern and western region. All three health centers are located in the central region of Uganda. District Y has a total population of about 2.000.000, of which roughly 1.370.000 live in the rural part of the district; district Z has 250.000 inhabitants in total, 200.000 living in the rural part; and district X finally counts 600.000 inhabitants with 440.000

---

9 I have changed the names of the districts for reasons of anonymity.

living in the rural areas (The State of Uganda Population Report 2016; figures are rounded). As mentioned before, two of the health centers had a functioning diabetes clinic once a week, and one facility offered testing and treatment for diabetes as part of the average outpatient medical services. District Y has seven bigger health facilities, District X two, and district Z has one[10]. This distribution may partially explain, why the numbers available of the individuals diagnosed with diabetes varies substantially between the districts.[11]

Located 16 km outside of Kampala in a north-westerly direction and a roughly 30 minutes car ride, district Y, was the closest health center from where I stayed in Kampala. Though a rather small health center – recently endorsed from a HC III to HC IV – this HC IV has a separate building for its diabetes clinic, unlike many other governmental health facilities (the hierarchy of health facilities will be explained in the next section). It is a small clinic with two rooms and a floor space of about 35 square meters. Enough space, however, for an examination room and a separate waiting room for the patients. The clinic took place once a week every Thursday between approximately 7.30 and 12.00 o'clock in the morning, depending on the number of patients. The head of the clinic, Sister Joy[12], whom we will meet again later in the empirical chapters, ran the hospital on her own. In contrast to the other health facilities I visited that had a large number of patients on a single clinic day, Sister Joy examined up to 20 patients on a diabetes clinic day. The diabetes clinic was initiated in 2007 and has ever since been run by Sister Joy. Inspired by a trip to Tanzania in 2009, where she received specialized training on diabetes care, Sister Joy started a diabetes association for her patients at the clinic. Collecting a yearly fee of 30.000 UGX[13] from her patients was and is a way to keep the clinic going even if the government fails to provide equipment and medicine.

The HC IV of district Z, 40 km and an hour's ride from Kampala on decent roads in western direction, too, has a diabetes clinic. The diabetes clinic was founded in the end of 2014. It runs every Monday from around 8 a.m. o'clock "until no patient is here anymore who needs to see me", like the responsible diabetes nurse, Sister Cathy said, which was often not before 5 p.m. She started working as a nurse in 1999, mainly in the outpatient department. Since "one year and eight months", she has now been working as a diabetes nurse after being trained "the essentials". Before that, she had never worked with diabetes patients, mainly because before

---

10 Based on the data from 2017. Therefore, the situation might have changed now.
11 The total number of individuals diagnosed with diabetes in district Z between 2011 and 2016 was 554, compared to a total number of 602 in district X and a total number of 3247 individuals with a diabetes diagnosis in district Y in the same time period.
12 Throughout the book, the term 'Sister' is used synonymous for nurse, since that is the term patients use and the way nurses refer to themselves. It does not indicate any kind of religious affiliation.
13 Approximately 8,20 US Dollars.

the clinic started, there was no equipment for testing. The name 'diabetes clinic' does not mean that the health center has an own building for it like it was the case in district Y. Instead, there is an examination room, which is reserved for the clinic every Monday and is otherwise used for the examination of patients in the outpatient department. The corridor in front of the room served as waiting area, at times endlessly congested with people waiting to be attended to. Sister Cathy at times saw up to 40 patients, a tiresome undertaking, considering that she had to document all the data into different books without assistance. Unlike Sister Joy, who tested her patients herself, Cathy sent her patients to the laboratory for testing.

This was also the case in the HC IV in district X, 28 km and about a one-hour ride eastbound of Kampala. Compared to the other two health facilities, it did not have a specialized diabetes clinic at the time I conducted my research, though there were plans of implementing one in the future. Like the district's health officer (DHO), Dr. Thomas said: "To be frank, we have not yet come far to NCDs [non-communicable diseases], but we are trying to work on it." This meant, that individuals would stand in line with all the other individuals who were waiting to be tested in the laboratory for various other diseases. This also meant, there was no specialized medical staff at the facility and since there was no diabetes association like in in the HC IV in district Y (at the time I was in Uganda, the HC IV in district Z was just planning to start an association too), the number of patients coming to be tested for diabetes remained zero for a long period of my fieldwork. The government had failed to procure medicine and testing strips for the glucometer for months. Individuals who needed glucose testing were therefore sent to nearby private health facilities if they could afford to pay the fees, or remained untested, untreated and unseen.

Sketching Uganda's health care system

The delivery of health care services is the backbone of a health system and offers one frame in which diabetes can be made visible by providing localities and a platform where diagnoses and testing can take place and care can be initiated. Yet as hinted at previously, not every health center offers services such as diagnostics or specialized clinics for individuals with diabetes in Uganda. Even where it could be expected, namely at the higher-level health facilities. Before moving on to the next chapter, I will briefly sketch out the main characteristics of Uganda's health care system[14]:

---

14 The data that can be found on e.g. the numbers of health care facilities within Uganda varies between different documents. To keep consistency, I will base my descriptions for this chapter

The biomedical health care system of Uganda consists of governmental/public[15] as well as private health facilities, whereby private health facilities can be divided into for-profit and not-for-profit health facilities (Lindelöw et al. 2003: 8). Uganda has no all citizens' health insurance scheme[16], but since March 2001 the user fees at all governmental health facilities have been abandoned - in theory. Medical consultations, diagnostics and treatment should be free of charge for everybody except in the private wings in governmental hospitals (Meessen et al. 2006: 2253; see also Men 2012). In practice, however, medical care does cost money very often even in governmental health facilities. I have met several diabetes patients who told me they would have to pay for their medication and the diagnostic tests, which meant that often times they would not be able to afford going to the hospital to receive treatment.

The health care system is, both in the governmental as well as in the private sector, structured in a hierarchical referral system staggered on seven levels: village health teams (VHT) are based on the lowest level, followed by health center II (HC II), health center III (HC III), health center IV (HC IV), general hospitals, regional hospitals and finally the national hospitals. The higher the level of the health center, the greater is usually the diversity and amount of services offered, resources and equipment available, and therefore the diagnostic and specialized care possibilities that can be offered at the facility. According to the Ministry of Health of Uganda (2014) there is a total of 5078 health facilities in the whole of Uganda. The majority of which are HC IIs, namely 3549. 1188 of the health facilities qualify as HC IIIs, 188 facilities are categorized as level HC IVs, 133 general hospitals, and 12 regional hospitals. The national referral hospitals stand at the top of the hierarchy, three in total in Uganda. They have the largest target population with 10 million people and are expected to provide highly specialized medical and surgical services. Furthermore, they are the institutions where medical research is conducted and training is offered for medical practitioners in various fields (MoH 2014).

---

mainly on the report "Uganda Hospital and Health Centre IV Census Survey, the first comprehensive assessment of availability of and capacity to offer health care services" in Uganda (MoH 2014: 3).

15 In the following I will use the term "governmental" instead of "public" facility, as this was the term mostly used by my informants.

16 I went to different private health insurance companies in Kampala just to find out a bit more about which services they offer and to whom. Besides the fact that it was hard to get information at all, most of them offered insurances only for companies or organizations. If they offered insurances for individuals, it was especially difficult to get insurance when having a chronic disease. Individuals with type 1 diabetes for instance will not be insured at all. Individuals with type 2 diabetes if at all, then only with a very high premium. As I was told by an insurance broker "it is the same when you get in a car accident and you go to the insurance the next day expecting them to pay". But she was not able to tell me what happened if an individual fell ill with diabetes while already being covered.

The services offered at the different levels can be summarized as follows:

Uganda has three levels of primary care facilities: level II (lower-level primary care facility), III (mid-level primary care facility) and IV (higher-level primary care facility) all focusing mainly on prevention and treatment of infectious illnesses. A level II primary care facility is the lowest level of formal health care delivery. It is mostly staffed by nurse aides and qualified nurses. A level III primary care facility has provisions for basic laboratory services, maternity care, and inpatient care (often for onward referral). It is usually staffed by nurse aides, qualified nurses and clinical officers (physician assistants). A level IV primary care facility is the level immediately below a district hospital and has a target population of 100,000 people. It has provisions for an operating theatre, in-patient and laboratory services, and is a referral facility for 20-30 level II and III primary care facilities under its jurisdiction. A level IV primary care facility is staffed by nurse aides, qualified nurses, clinical officers and doctors, although the majority does not have doctors. (MoH 2014: 35)

As mentioned, Uganda's health care system functions on a referral basis. Meaning if a lower level health facility is not able to handle a disease or provide the needed care, an individual will be referred to the next higher-level facility until the facility offers the services, care and treatment required to manage the disease. The scope of duties at lower health facilities, HC II and HC III, mainly evolves around the diagnosis and treatment of medicable infectious diseases, including the flue, malaria, pneumonia, and urinary tract infections. The increasing availability of different rapid diagnostic tests for diseases, which were usually handled at higher health facilities with more complex laboratory equipment, for instance HIV or hepatitis, has facilitated the application of these tests also at lower health facilities (Umlauf 2017).

The descriptions so far depict the ideal case. In practice, the referral system and the services offered at each level health facility are not always functioning according to their scale. This holds true for infectious diseases, but especially for chronic disease like diabetes, where symptoms of diabetes have to be recognized as such in the first place. The glucometer can aid and confirm diagnoses. Further, the glucometer is a point-of-care device, which can be used also in settings where a laboratory is absent, such as at lower health facilities in Uganda, it can rarely be found in governmental health facilities lower than HC IV. Like I was told by an employee of the Ministry of Health responsible for the procurement of medical technologies:

"Now, those glucometers we have. They are there in the districts. But sometimes it is a challenge where to find them and that makes referral complicated, because where should they refer the patients if they cannot be sure the device is there in the other facility? Diabetes has been one of the diseases, which has not been top in terms of ranking when they do the surveys to see the prevalence and all that. Diabetes has not been a big issue until recently. That is why I would say at all hospitals you would get glucometers and some HCIVs. HCIIIs I don't think so."

In Uganda's health care system, which is characterized by underfunded and weak health infrastructures, guidelines and regulations for diabetes care, including the handling of glucometers, are still missing. Diabetes care in governmental health facilities remains haphazardly available. While health care is said to be free in Uganda, especially individuals with diabetes face costs when seeking care: stock outs of medication, including oral agents and insulin for the treatment of diabetes, and absent testing equipment frequently requires individuals to pay for their treatment and testing at private facilities and pharmacies. Contrary to government policy, some governmental facilities often only test and provide medication against a fee in the face of resource deficiencies.

A roadmap to visibility – outline of the book

The book you are about to read comprises seven central chapters, nestled between this introductory part and concluding remarks. Hereby each chapter intends to shed light on a different aspect, which either contributes to or hampers the visibility, perceptibility and the making of diabetes on different levels and by diverse actors. Since each of the chapters has its own theoretical introduction and argument, each chapter can be read independently of one another. At the same time the overall picture expands and becomes more nuanced the more chapters you decide to read. The more of this book you will read, the more you will delve into the complexities and entanglements of diabetes. The more you will read, the more you will understand the diagnostics of diabetes and what contributes to the struggle for its visibility and its making.

The next chapter intends triple-fold: firstly, diabetes will be defined from a biomedical perspective, staging this disease as a chronic condition without prospects of cure and without a predictable course of disease. The longevity of the disease has consequences for its understanding as well as for the provision of resources and care. Secondly, you will be taken on a medical journey from past to present understandings and perceptions of diabetes, and its transformation: from a formerly mysterious, puzzling and deadly disease into a chronic condition achieved through technological intervention and progress and advanced knowledge. On the flipside, the (hi)story of diabetes as it is noted down in textbooks is a strikingly localized disease where hardly anything can be found on the history of diabetes in the majority world. This in turn may explain the invisibility of this disease in contexts such as Uganda and why diabetes can repeatedly be reframed as a "new" and "unseen" disease. Finally, chapter one will outline some of the diagnostic possibilities there are to diagnose diabetes including recommendations and (contested) diagnostic thresholds.

Diabetes is not a disease, which transcends national borders. It is not a disease that endangers the health of the global public the way infectious diseases do. I therefore suggest that non-communicable diseases are caught in a vortex of suspense provoked by the rigidity and partially inflexibility of the regimes of global health in this 21st century, which is dedicated to global health security and humanitarian biomedicine. Though global health intends to improve the health outcomes on a global scale, it might be at the expense of conditions that do not fall in either of these two categories. As a possible result, global actions are only slowly taken up and donor funding of any kind is pending, local policies and guidelines remain stagnant. Further the lack of comprehensive numerical data is one major reason for why diabetes receives little attention in Uganda's health care system and beyond. Different types of evidence, such as narratives and ethnographic evidence, or "real-life evidence" as an informant once called it, then become ever more important to make diabetes, and the individuals who are affected by it, seen.

Subsequently, chapter three lays the conceptual fundament on which the empirical material for this book is built. I propose to look at diabetes and its making through the conceptual lenses of evidence-based medicine, (health) infrastructures and translation. By linking these different concepts to the study of diabetes – and to one technological object, the glucometer – I want to picture how diverse actors engage in its use and how each different practice brings about a different kind of knowledge and visibility. Whereas the technologies travel 'borderless', the borders they might face are the borders created for instance by the rigidity of other technologies, such as evidence-based medicine, as well as the borders built by weak health infrastructures and resource shortages that limit the radius of operation.

Starting from chapter four up until chapter seven we will immerse ourselves in the empirical body of this book. As hinted at before, in each of these chapters we will encounter the glucometer – sometimes more explicit, sometimes less explicit – as strikingly multidimensional actor: it will present itself as a tool to deliver (numerical and epidemiological) evidence contributing to the prevalence rates of diabetes in Uganda. It will be the diagnostic device producing and revealing more individuals who will then be labeled "diabetic". I will appear as a contradictory object that limits uncertainty, while it is at the same time being the source that creates this uncertainty. The beauty but also the curse of this technology is neither dependent on a predefined group of people who may engage in its use, nor is it bound to a specific locality, we will find ourselves in health centers and laboratories, in people's homes, on a roadside or in a primary school. No matter where we will find ourselves and who the actors are we will come to meet, they all in one way or the other, with one intention or another, make diabetes and related aspects of it visible. The conclusion, finally, will offer a platform to discuss the main findings of this book.

Before we proceed, a final note: the names of the individuals you will come to meet are aliases. As mentioned I have also changed the names of the districts in which I have worked. I have, however, retained the names of organizations. Further I have, where suitable, merged several occurrences or interviews into a single one to ease the readability and avoid confusing enumerations. I have hereby not changed the content. Finally, I am well aware that I have made many certain choices throughout this book. I have for instance chosen which stories to include or to exclude, or I have decided in which way I would like to retell them and the wording I use thereby. I know there are other stories I could have told, there are different conceptual paths I could have taken, other references I could have included. There is always something you could have done differently afterwards. Nevertheless, if Geertz, as he is quoted by Wendland (2010), was right and the true purpose of anthropology is to increase the number of stories out there, then we may simply read the following book as *one* possible story about glucometers and the making of diabetes in Uganda (Wendland 2010: 221). A story told from the vantage point of a small device, the disease it renders visible and about the people who use it.

1. "If you are lacking insulin" – Diabetes Mellitus

> If you're lacking insulin
> You must act accordingly,
> For, alas, it is Man's fate
> That his innards often fail.
> Truly, though it is not too late,
> Diet is the magic word
> To embellish all your days
> You must kick the sugar ways [...]
> You'll achieve 'most any goal
> If your guide is self-control.
> You will stay both trim and slim,
> Avoid sickness, thank the Lord,
> Watch the fatties jealous looks
> At your meagre calories.
> Where there's a lack of insulin
> The best help is self-discipline [...]
> ——Wilhelm Jaenecke 1969

Perhaps you feel similar like I did when I, for the first time, started working on and with diabetes for my master's project in 2012. You might be wondering what diabetes is other than a disease *somehow* related to sugar or (too high) body weight. Where does diabetes come from? Diabetes is a disease many of us have heard about. You might have relatives or friends who have it and will know a bit more. But perhaps you have never been confronted with anybody who has this disease. In this case, diabetes may indeed be a disease that has to do with sugar and body weight somehow. What is diabetes? Without lying claim to offer a full account of what diabetes *is*, this chapter aims at giving an overview of diabetes. For if we deal with this disease, there are some things we ought to know: what the symptoms are, what happens in and to our body if we have diabetes and how it can be diagnosed and treated. Those are some aspects I hope to give you an answer to. I would now like to take you along on the journey of a formerly deadly disease making its way to a chronic condition.

The abstract of the poem "The clever diabetic" (1969) gives us a clue of what diabetes can deal with: insulin, diet, (eating no) sugar, self-control, (over-)weight and (lack of?)[1] self-discipline. Those are some facets we can relate to it. But there is more; diabetes goes beyond its mere medical manifestations, as Engelhardt states "diabetes is both a medical and a cultural topic; disease is never just an objective phenomenon, but always involves a suffering human body and being who possesses awareness and speech, lives in a social setting and adopts an attitude to this disease" (Engelhardt 1989: 6). As we will see, it is a disease that comes into being and gets a name and shape through technology. Therefore, it is a disease that has a fascinating (hi)story: it is a disease that can tell us something about the quest for control over disease, about the miracles (medical) technologies promise and how these technologies influence the perception and handling of disease.

Not just about sugar

Before we continue to dig deeper into the (hi)story of diabetes, let us have a go at defining diabetes on a biomedical level. The first important aspect of diabetes is that there is not only *one* type of diabetes, but there are different types of it. Diabetes is often distinguished between three major forms: type 1 diabetes, type 2 diabetes and gestational diabetes. As my empirical material is mainly based on type 2, little on type 1[2] and not at all on gestational diabetes, I will not talk about gestational diabetes here and instead focus on the first two types[3].

Diabetes type 1 used to be known as "juvenile diabetes" or "insulin-dependent" diabetes. It was called juvenile diabetes, because it usually occurs in young children or teenagers. Insulin-dependent diabetes, because individuals having this type rely on insulin for survival. Though the cause is not yet fully understood, diabetes type 1 is thought of being an autoimmune reaction where the pancreatic cells that are

---

1 There is the prevailing assumption that especially type 2 diabetes is the result of an individual's lack of discipline and self-control, overeating and living sedentary life-styles. Though this perception might hold true for some examples on a very superficial level, it is an oversimplified perception that ignores the reality and life-worlds of these individuals. Reynolds Whyte adds for consideration that these life-styles may rather be imposed than actively chosen for why the term life condition seems more appropriate in this context (Reynolds Whyte 2012; 2014b).
2 The reason why I hardly have cases of individuals with type 1 diabetes is because many clinics in Uganda do not (yet) distinguish between type 1 and type 2 diabetes. In fact, from the three clinics where I conducted extensive fieldwork, only one was offering separate services for type 1 and type 2 diabetes. Further both types are hard to distinguish, as they require high-tech lab tests for differentiation (WHO 2016a: 26).
3 For those interested in gestational diabetes, a type of diabetes occurring during pregnancy, Seshia (2015) and Smith-Morris (2005) offer a great introduction.

responsible for producing insulin are destroyed. Since diabetes type 2 usually affects adults at the prime of their economic life, it has been called "adult-onset" or "non-insulin-dependent" diabetes. Unlike type 1 diabetes, type 2 diabetes is not a result of too little or a total lack of insulin, but rather the body's incapability to react appropriately to the insulin signal.[4] Either or, diabetes is a complex metabolic disorder and physicians study years, and have to prove themselves in clinical practice in order to learn how to take care of individuals having this condition. Expertise in the field of diabetes does not prevent physicians and other experts from continuously debating and controverting about this disease, especially when it comes to nutrition (what to eat and not to eat), medication practices (especially when it comes to type 2 diabetes), but also concerning the classification and diagnosis of the disease (what are appropriate cut-off values of a normal/abnormal blood glucose level). We will have a closer look at this shortly.

The following pages are for those of you, who know little about diabetes and I hope I can offer somewhat of an overview in an understandable way. That is, squeeze a very complex disease into rather simple words.[5] But before you continue to read, there is one thing about diabetes that we should all memorize. To say it with the words of Feudtner: "The key point to remember is that diabetes mellitus is not just about sugar" (Feudtner 2003: xix). To be able to understand diabetes, we have to know how a *healthy* body metabolizes food. When we eat, we digest the food in our stomachs and bowels into its different elements including fats (lipids), proteins (amino acids) and carbohydrates (starches and sugars such as glucose). Our body, respectively our organs are able to decide how to use these different elements once they have entered our bloodstream. Feudtner describes the process the following: "[Elements have four fates], they are burned immediately as fuel, incorporated into the structure of the body, converted into other basic elements, or stored away for later use. Between the meals, the same organs direct the retrieval of the stored food. The decision of how the digested or stored food will be used is, in a manner of speaking, determined by a committee, which we might call the Council of Food Utilization" (Feudtner 2003: xix). What Feudtner terms the Council of Food Utilization is basically the compilation of our different organs such as the thyroid for example, the liver, our muscles and brain, or of course the organ that interests us most at the moment: the pancreas. The pancreas consists of specialized cells

---

4 The terms insulin-dependent diabetes mellitus (IDDM) and non-insulin dependent diabetes mellitus (NIDDM) have expressly been dismissed after a consensus of the WHO in 2000 stating that these terms would too much focus on the treatment of diabetes rather than the underlying mechanisms behind it (Kerner et al. 2001: 14). Further the terms miss out, that also in type 2 diabetes there are individuals who may require insulin and that type 2 diabetes is increasingly affecting children and young adults.
5 I apologize to all the (diabetes) experts among you for my allegedly oversimplified terms to describe this complex disease.

called alpha (α), beta (β) and delta (δ) cells and can be found in the small clusters called the islets of Langerhans (ibid.).

Whereas our brain freely utilizes the amount of glucose it needs for its functions, as well as our muscles use as much glucose they need when we for instance exercise, other organs cannot freely utilize glucose or other elements liberally. When it comes to the decision on which organ may use which element, our organs will have to "communicate with each other via the language of hormones" (Feudtner 2003: xx). Every organ has its own hormonal depository. These hormones are employed to send information across and within our body. Our organs continuously discuss and coordinate how to best use the food we have eaten, as well as what and how much food we need in order to keep our body going: do we for example need the food for growing, thinking or to fill up our depositories?

The most important organ when it comes to diabetes is, as mentioned before, the pancreas. More specifically, the pancreas and the β cells. The β cells are responsible to oversee how much dietary energy is circulating in our blood. When the digested food is traveling through our body, the β cells will notify our tissues that our blood is rich in nutrient energy. This is possible, because the β cells release the hormone insulin into our blood circulation, which is used to transport this information.[6] As soon as the hormone insulin has passed on this information, our body, or our tissues to be precise, can start to occlude the nutrients from our blood and either transform them into energy, or stock them in the respective depository. Diabetes will then occur when the hormone insulin is not able to pass on the information properly or fails completely to do so (ibid.). There are different causes as to why insulin fails to manage its purpose and to understand these reasons we have to get back to the former distinction between type 1 diabetes and type 2 diabetes:

Type 1 diabetes is characterized by a destruction of the β cells caused by the immune system leading to a collapse in the release of insulin. There are different explanations and opinions for why this collapse emerges – a disparity of opinions leading from genes as the causal factors for diabetes to viruses as causal agent – but the important information for us is that when the β cells do not convey the message to the body that the blood is enriched with nutrients, our body will always think it needs more food, even if we have eaten enormous amounts. As Feudtner explains, "[l]acking any insulin, the well-fed metabolism behaves paradoxically, as though the body is being starved. This starvation metabolism fails to take sugar that is in the blood and either burn it as fuel or store it away" (Feudtner 2003: xxi). Without insulin, sugar will amass in our blood stream leading to increased glucose levels, a condition referred to as *hyperglycemia*.

---

6 Insulin is only among many hormones involved in these processes; but it is the one that interests us most when it comes to diabetes.

The situation is a bit different for individuals with type 2 diabetes. Instead of failing to convey the message that our blood is circulating a lot of food energy, the message transported by insulin is "ignored" by the tissues, it is not read properly. In this type, there is not a lack of insulin, but instead a surplus of insulin every time someone eats. This communication error becomes a problem as soon as the β cells are no longer able to keep up the massive amount of insulin that now has to be produced to come up for this error; the body receives too much food compared to the amount of insulin the β cells are able to produce. Although in type 2 diabetes the body does not have a problem with a lack of insulin but instead too much insulin, the glucose in the blood cannot be extracted and therefore too leads to elevated blood sugar levels, to hyperglycemia (ibid.). *Hypoglycemia* in contrast relates to a too low blood sugar level. It arises for instance when an individual has injected too much insulin or has eaten too little. It is the most acute complication of diabetes mellitus, as a too low blood sugar may impair the brain and cardiac functions. If the glucose levels drop amply, the individual's cognitive functions will be disturbed (Evans and Amiel 2002). This is why it is hypoglycemia, which patients often fear the most, as we will also see later in the empirical chapters.

Before we proceed, let us recapitulate some few aspects. We will focus on two major types of diabetes: Type 1 diabetes and type 2 diabetes. What both types have in common is a condition called hyperglycemia, which means elevated blood sugar levels. The problematic issue for an individual with diabetes is that the body contains too much blood sugar in relation to the amount of insulin delivered by the pancreas. The blood sugar levels will either rise if our body cannot produce enough insulin to match up to the amount of sugar in the bloodstream, or if the pancreas fails to produce insulin. If this state of elevated blood sugar levels in our blood persists, we develop diabetes. Summarized and put into one sentence: we develop diabetes if our blood sugar levels are continuously elevated resulting from either too little insulin produced or a total failure to produce insulin (Kerner et al. 2001; see also Alberti and Zimmet 1998). Though the origination process of diabetes in type 1 and type 2 diabetes differs, the symptoms of type 1 and type 2 diabetes are nearly the same. Nonetheless, it is the second type where the disease comes silently, mantled in insidious symptoms and often leaves an individual undiagnosed until severe complications have developed; and it is the second type that makes the vast majority of diabetes cases worldwide, about 90-95% (ADA 2016: 16). This insidious onset of diabetes, leaving a diagnosis until late in the progression of the disease, has brought along the sobriquet "the silent killer". It does not kill suddenly, but gradually.

Ascribing a type of diabetes to an individual, whether type 1 diabetes (which was usually referred to affecting children and youth) and type 2 diabetes (usually diagnosed in adults) is no longer as easy. The American Diabetes Association (ADA) states that "assigning a type of diabetes to an individual often depends on the circumstances present at the time of diagnosis, with individuals not necessarily fitting clearly into a single category [...]. Some patients cannot be clearly classified as having type 1 or type 2 diabetes [...]. The traditional paradigms of type 2 diabetes occurring only in adults and type 1 diabetes only in children are no longer accurate, as both diseases occur in both cohorts" (ADA 2015: S8).

However, the resulting high level of blood sugar can lead to all sorts of havoc in both types. The overflow of blood sugar into the urine causes the patient to urinate copiously (polyuria), which in turn makes the patient extremely thirsty, creating an urge to drink excessively (polydipsia). In addition, without insulin present, the metabolism also mishandles the storage of proteins and fats. All these effects leave the patient with a ravenous appetite (polyphagia) and, over years, at great risk for various medical complications. The reduced blood flow increases the likelihood of developing neuropathy, a damage of the nerves, which in turn encourages infections of the limbs with the potential need of amputation due to gangrene such as the diabetic foot (Morrish et al. 2001). When the small blood vessels in the retina are damaged over time, this can lead to blindness, the so-called diabetic retinopathy. A patient with diabetes is more likely to develop a cardiovascular disease, kidney failure and is apoplectic, meaning prone to suffer a stroke. Generally, the risk of dying is 50% higher in diabetes patients compared to people of the same age who are healthy (Roglic et al. 2005: 2133). Diabetes treatment consists of lowering the blood sugar levels either with oral agents (hypoglycemics) in the case of type 2 diabetes; or insulin for individuals with type 1 diabetes as well as individuals with type 2 diabetes, where an oral agent is ineffective.

Both types of diabetes are deadly if left untreated, and patients with either form are susceptible to complications even if the disease is treated properly. This at least is how we understand the disease today: a chronic metabolic disorder, requiring life-long treatment and regular medical surveillance, including self-monitoring practices. But it was a long way until we reached the point of understanding we have today, and we have not yet reached the end of it. The following section will take you on a brief journey through time in the (hi)story of diabetes and its way from a former deadly to a chronic disease.

The mysterious illness: one (hi)story of diabetes

History is never only a consecution of events, but it is always a story, a narrative that is being conveyed through the lived experience of the individuals that are part of the story and constitute it. Diabetes has been occupying people's minds for a long time and has made its mark also in literature and art, inspiring poets and novelists alike[7]. The poem you read in the beginning of this chapter "The clever Diabetic" by Jaenecke (1969) is one example. The German writer Thomas Mann is for instance another, who, in his novel *Buddenbrooks* (1901), lets one of his characters, senator James Möllendorf, suffer from diabetes describing that "[t]he instincts of self-preservation were so far absent in this old man that in the last years of his life he increasingly succumbed to a passion for cakes and pastry [until] he was found lifeless, his mouth still full of half-chewed cake" (Mann 1901, as cited in Engelhardt 1989: 10). The past offers us numerous examples of individuals who allegedly had diabetes (though it is hard to be certain retrospectively whether it was really diabetes in all cases): for instance, the Polish King, Michal Korybut Wisniowiecki (1640–1673); the Saxon King, August the Great (1670–1733); the painter Paul Cézanne (1839–1906) or the composer Giacomo Puccini (1858–1924), whose opera "Madame Butterfly" was jestingly termed the "Diabetic's Opera" (Engelhardt 1989: 7f).

You may wonder why we should look at the history of diabetes, if we are ultimately trying to grasp its impacts in the present? One of the more obvious reasons is that if we look at the history of diabetes, we can see how the strong will for medical and technological progress has metamorphosed a formerly deadly disease into the chronic condition it is today. Another reason is that we might be able to understand or at least illuminate the paradox, or "ironic dilemma" as Feudtner termed it, "created by our prevailing views of illness and medicine, personal responsibility, and the pursuit of control over disease" (Feudtner 2003: 4). A dilemma, we will also be confronted with again later in this book. Without wanting to reveal too much in advance, the history of diabetes is not only a story of medical progress when it comes to understanding disease from a biomedical perspective. Furthermore, it is story it of technological invention, innovation and progress. There is even more to it: you will come to realize that the (hi)story of diabetes has been a strikingly "Western" (hi)story in the past and often continues to be pictured as such even in the present. This will have important implications for when we look at diabetes as a global issue and phenomenon in the following chapter. But for now, let us have a look at the history of diabetes.

Diabetes has been puzzling medical authors for over three millennia. If we could turn back the hands of time, far back until 81–138 B.C, we could have possibly met a Greek physician named Aretaeus of Cappadocia, who was practicing in Rome and Alexandria. In his treatise "On the Causes and Indications of Acute and Chronic Diseases" his observations made then are mostly still valid today. He wrote:

> Diabetes is a dreadful affliction, not very frequent among men, being a melting down of the flesh and limbs into urine. The patients never stop making water and

---

7 An entry point to an expansive medical and cultural history of diabetes is offered by e.g. Dietrich von Engelhardt (1989).

the flow is incessant, like the opening of the aqueducts. Life is short, unpleasant and painful, thirst unquenchable, drinking excessive and disproportionate to the large quantity of urine, for yet more urine is passed [...]. If for a while they abstain from drinking, their mouths become parched and their bodies dry; the viscera seem scorched up, the patients are affected by nausea, restlessness and a burning thirst, and within a short time they expire. (Aretaeus, as cited in Medvei 1993: 34, 37)

There was earlier mention of a disease with diabetes-like symptoms in the *Papyrus Ebers*[8], where a "too great emptying of the urine" was described suggesting a treatment using wheat grains, fruit, and sweet beer (Poretsky et al. 2010: 3). Yet Aretaeus is thought of being the first offering an expansive portrayal of the symptoms of this "new" and puzzling disease. An acute illness or a stomach disease, followed by a poisoning of the kidneys and the bladder would be the underlying causes for this suffering, Aretaeus reasoned, proposing a mild diet and steam baths as treatment options (Engelhardt 1989: 3). Etymologically the term diabetes derives from the Greek, meaning siphon as in 'traverse or flow through' – relating to the frequent urination as one of the main symptoms of diabetes. Aretaeus explained "that is the reason, I believe, why the sickness has been called diabetes, as if it were a wine siphon, because liquid is not retained in the body but uses the human being like a tube through which it can drain itself off" (Aretaeus, as cited in Schadewaldt 1989: 45). Aretaeus and his contemporary, the renowned Roman physician Galen, considered diabetes a rare disease. Galen attributed the development of diabetes to a weakness of the kidney and named it "diarrhea of the urine" (Poretsky et al. 2010: 3).

Between 400 and 500 B.C. the Indian physicians Charak and Sushrut were possibly the first to describe the sweetness of the urine naming it "madhumeha", honey urine, and the first who distinguished between two types of diabetes (Zimmet et al. 2002: 1635). They noticed that individuals being small in physique developed diabetes at an earlier age compared to individuals of sturdy build, who were usually older and lived longer after the onset of diabetes. It is them who can be seen as the pioneers when it comes to testing diabetes, as they related the sweet urine of a person with diabetes to the attraction of flies and ants[9] (Poretsky et al. 2010: 3).

During his travels the Spanish Talmudic scholar and physician Maimonides, who lived in Egypt most of his life (1135–1204), noted that he had hardly heard of

---

8 The Papyrus Ebers is the oldest medical text from the sixteenth century B.C., which was found at Luxor in Egypt in 1872 in an ancient grave in Thebes and is "considered to be the first allusion about diabetes mellitus in the history of medicine" (Papaspyros 1964: 4).
9 To test whether ants and flies are attracted by urine is a technique, which is occasionally still used today by some individuals for instance in Tanzania or Uganda (Nnko et al. 2015; Reynolds Whyte 2012).

diabetes occurring in 'cold' Europe whereas it was often observed in 'warm' Africa: "I, too, did not see it [diabetes] in the West [Spain and/or Morocco], nor did any of the teachers under whom I studied, mention that they had seen it. However here in Egypt, in the course of approximately ten years, I have seen more than twenty people who suffered from this illness. This leads to the conclusion that this illness occurs mostly in warm countries. Perhaps the waters of the Nile, because of their sweetness, may play a role in this" (Maimonides aphorism 69, as cited in Rosner 1997: 52–53).[10]

The list of physicians and people who set their wits to diabetes could be continued; a list of people searching for clues, answers and explanations for the origin and treatment of this puzzling disease. The basis, however, for how we understand certain aspects of diabetes today, can be attributed to discoveries between the 16th and 18th century in Europe. In the beginning of the 16th century the Swiss physician Aureolus Theophrastus Bombastus von Hohenheim, more commonly known as Paracelsus, detected a white substance after the urine of his patients with diabetes had vaporized. He then thought that this white substance was salt and inferred that the excessive thirst and urination that was plaguing these individuals was due to a salt residue in the kidneys (Medvei 1993: 55), a hypothesis that was falsified a century later.

In 1674, the Englishman Thomas Willis published "The Diabetes or Pissing Evil". Like many physicians before him, Willis was greatly impressed by the volume of urine that people with diabetes produced, observing that "those laboring with this Disease, piss a great deal more than they drink, or take of any liquid aliment; and moreover, they have always joined with its continual thirst, and a gentle, and as it were hectic Fever" (Feudtner 2003: 5). "Experiments and Observations on the Urine in Diabetics", was the title of the book of Matthew Dobson, who in 1776 identified the sweet-tasting substance in the urine as sugar – a turning point in the history of diabetes (but it took another 86 years until the sugar was determined as glucose, the precursor for later early urine tests as we will see). He created a theory, which related diabetes to the whole body rather than to a problem of the kidneys, like many before him had thought (Poretsky et al. 2010: 4). Shortly after Dobson, in 1788, for the first time a connection was drawn between the pancreas and the development of diabetes when a physician, Thomas Cawley, noticed that his patients with pancreatic injuries eventually developed diabetes (ibid.).

Though the sweetness of urine was already documented in the beginning of the first millennium, the adjunct *mellitus* (Latin for 'treacly or sweet as honey')

---

10 This observation, respectively this assumption, did not hold true and today the development of diabetes is surely not related to the climate but is said to be related especially to lifestyle. However, what fascinated me about Maimonides assumption was that this is the only relation between diabetes and the African continent I could find during my entire research.

was added by the surgeon general to the British Army, John Rollo, not before the late 18th century.[11] Rollo suggested an "animal diet" as dietary therapy for diabetes: blood pudding, rancid meats and a combination of milk and limewater – endeavors to find a dietary solution that the bodies of people with diabetes could adapt to (Feudtner 2003: 6). However, all attempts to stave off death with complex dietary regimens failed. Children did not live longer than three years after their diagnosis, adults above 60 years of age no longer than six years. Even if a patient could afford the best possible medical care, life was contingent on dietary therapies, ravaged by infections, ending in coma or starvation: the diagnosis of diabetes was a death sentence (ibid.).

While for millennia the cause of, and treatment for, this mysterious disease continued to be opaque, the fate of individuals with diabetes was to change when insulin was discovered in the summer of 1921 at the University of Toronto by Frederick G. Banting, Charles H. Best, John J.R. Macleod and other researchers – the greatest turning point in the biography of diabetes, and a discovery, for which Banting and Macleod received the Nobel Prize two years later in 1923. One year after the commercial production of insulin was already on the way.[12] The news of the discovery of insulin spread like a wildfire and doctors and patients raised new hopes that a cure had been found for this fatal disease. Newspapers spurred on these hopes: the New York Times published a newspaper article in May 1923 entitled "Diabetes, Dread Disease, Yields to New Gland Cure" reporting how "one by one, the implacable enemies of man, the diseases which seek his destruction, are overcome by science" (Feudtner 2003: 8). The message, which now was transported, was that insulin worked wonders – a magic bullet had been found. Pictures circulated of children half starved, nothing but skin and bones before the treatment of insulin and then, the same children after the treatment with insulin, having chubby cheeks and a big smile on their face (ibid.). The daughter of the then Minister of Foreign Affairs, Elizabeth Hughes, was one of the first children to receive and profit from insulin injections and was considered to be "practically cured". Robert Lansing, a great politician who also suffered from diabetes "gained greatly in flesh and in strength [...] his dietary restrictions have been completely removed, so that he is permitted to eat as much as he desires of all varieties of food" (ibid.). The news that was spread was that the battle against diabetes had been won with the invention of insulin. In 1930, the diabetes expert Frederick Allen proclaimed, "[d]iabetes has

---

11 The adjunct diabetes mellitus also helped to distinguish this condition from diabetes insipidus. It is not necessary here to go into detail on diabetes insipidus; in short: it is a very uncommon condition and not related to blood sugar. It is a disease, in which the kidneys fail to prevent the flux of water (Engelhardt 1989).

12 For those interested in a more detailed and expansive description of the discovery of insulin, Michael Bliss (2007) offers a detailed insight in his book "The discovery of insulin".

been scientifically mastered. Theoretically, every patient can be expected to live out his full natural lifetime" (Feudtner 2003: 9).

The (hi)story of diabetes is a "symbol of scientific progress and the prospect of human mastery over disease" (Feudtner 2003: 10). Though in theory the discovery of insulin "as a heroic wonder drug to rescue patients, vanquish disease [and] banish suffering" (ibid.) indeed changed the lives of many individuals with diabetes, insulin had not only solved problems, but it had created new ones. The success stories that could be read around the time of the insulin discovery whitewashed the fact that access to insulin was reserved for those, who could afford this expensive treatment and who had access to this new knowledge in the first place. Not every doctor especially in the beginning of the 1920s knew about the new discovery that had been made in the laboratories of Toronto. There were, and today still are, patients with diabetes who on the one hand never knew they had the disease. On the other hand, many of them did and do not have access to medical treatment. For all those individuals, diabetes continued to be a death sentence, or a death in installments.

Obscured by the success story that insulin had brought along, the realities of the people who were living with diabetes were largely left unseen. As Feudtner states, emphasizing this

> miraculous event, these accounts ignore the more sober legacy of this "miracle" – all the problems that remained, all the new problems created by the transmutation of diabetes into a chronic disease. Exulting in an unexamined belief in progress, they fail to grapple with the difficult task of weighing the mixed consequences of medical intervention – all the years of life added poised against all the ramifications of living with a chronic, often debilitating disease. (ibid.)

And another aspect that becomes apparent when looking at the (hi)story of diabetes is that all people that found their way into the story in one way or another have one thing in common: they were people of affluence, wealthy people or at least moving in the upper-class circles of their time. Intractable even today is the perception that diabetes is a disease of the wealthy, the rich who can afford an effusive lifestyle with good food and drinks, or as many people in Uganda would say, diabetes is a disease for the White and a disease for the rich.

A disease without (hi)story?

Perhaps it was naïve to think that I will be able to get some details on the history of diabetes in Uganda. Was it naïve? Perhaps it was a rather optimistic attitude to assume that there have to be numbers written down anywhere, somewhere in an archive in Uganda, in some document, wherever. Numbers or documents that reveal when the first cases of diabetes were noted and how at that time diabetes was diagnosed and treated. When was it really that the numbers of people with diabetes were increasing? When was it that diabetes started to emerge to a public health problem in Uganda? Though it would most likely be possible to get at least a clue or somewhat of an answer for this last question by combing through different documents and climbing the back of recent discourses, it became clear quite fast that there was no (hi)story of diabetes in Uganda before say the 1980s or even later. Hardly any evidence or proof that this disease actually existed there (possibly the same holds true for many other countries in sub-Saharan Africa). But I do remember very well how much hope I had when I met one of Uganda's few (there are about three in total) diabetologists in his doctor's office in Kampala. He told me that the oldest reference that could be found was an article published in the Journal of Tropical Hygiene written by a guy, who today is called the father of modern medicine in Uganda: Sir Albert Cook, a doctor from Great Britain traveling to Uganda as a missionary back in 1901. What he wrote in this article was that diabetes as well as hypertension was extremely rare in "the African"[13]. Though not very cogent, there at least is tiny evidence of diabetes. At that time, it was known that if the urine would attract insects, this meant that there was sugar in the urine and this person could be diabetic, the diabetologist explained. But other than that, he had no idea. Naturally it is nearly impossible to track down evidence of a disease if there is no documentation anywhere. Before 1988 there was no formal way of dealing with diabetes, there were no records, the expert told me.

When I spoke to the program manager of non-communicable diseases (NCDs) at the Ministry of Health she said that it was simply weird to look at diabetes in the 1980s. During her training as a medical doctor she indeed learned about diabetes but it was taught that it was only common in Western people because of their high economy. Consequently, it was not taken seriously and what she had learned about diabetes until then was soon forgotten. How, I wonder, should people remember or think about seemingly unimportant diseases like diabetes (that only concern the wealthy anyway) when since the 1980s Uganda and the HIV epidemic[14] that struck it hard filled the headlines of newspapers, radio reports, the news internationally as well as it fueled global health concerns? It is a dead end to try to understand or get a picture of the history of diabetes in Uganda, but nevertheless, it leaves us with a critical stance. Not everything that big players in global health postulate holds true, especially then, when their claims (of evidence) are not (sufficiently) followed by action. How can a disease be recognized as a threatening disease, if it has no story to relate to? Innumerable new technologies traveling far distances,

---

13 Unfortunately, I was not able to access this article the diabetologist mentioned and therefore relied on what he could remember from when he himself had read it during his studies.
14 See Kuhanen (2008) for an overview of the HIV/AIDS epidemic in Uganda.

but what they cannot bring back are lost or forgotten histories, they can only write new histories.

While during the lifetime of Aretaeus diabetes was "not at all frequent in humans" (Schadewaldt 1989: 43), the situation has changed significantly since then. In 2014, the number of diabetics worldwide has reached an estimated number of 422 million and diabetes was the cause of 1.5 million deaths of adults aged 18 and above (the actual figures as suspected to be much higher) – compared to an estimation of 627.000 deaths due to malaria in the same year (WHO 2016b). In 2010, 3.4 million people died as a consequence of an overly high blood sugar level. However, besides the number of deaths, there is in fact a big difference between diabetes and malaria: malaria occurs exclusively in malaria-endemic countries, diabetes can occur everywhere, in any-*body*. "Gone are the times when NCDs were 'diseases of affluence' and only of industrialized countries" (Puska 2011: 269), as now around 75% of diabetes affect people living in low-and middle-income countries (IDF 2015).

Is it true what Hjelm and Atwine (2011) state, that the diabetes pandemic is "related to urbanization with longevity and changes of lifestyle, from a traditional active way of life to a modern sedentary style with unhealthy diets and obesity, combined with genetic susceptibility development and probably also poverty" (Hjelm and Atwine 2011: 1)? This assumption is widely acknowledged. But technology holds a great share in this diabetes pandemic as well: diagnostic technology is the means to reveal and categorize disease; and it is the means to *make* diabetes patients. How the diagnostic possibilities have developed over time, from where it started and where we are today will be the core of the following sections.

From urine to blood

Diagnostics are the core when it comes to identifying and uncovering disease. As a laboratory technician in Uganda once said, "diagnostics are the glasses through which diseases become apparent and visible." Later in this book, we will have a closer look at exactly this essential moment in the disease-(hi)story of a person with diabetes and the (re)assuring encounter between medical practitioner and patient. As we have gone through a brief (hi)story of diabetes, we will now turn to the possibilities that have emerged over time to test and diagnose the disease. The path will take us along from first sugar screenings with (simple) urine tests followed by rather complex reagent strip systems to monitor the glucose in the blood. Though I do not aim at outlining the history of the technological advancements' diagnosis of diabetes in detail, there are some interesting developments in the course of time, which are worth mentioning.

That it was a long way from the early beginnings of diabetes diagnostics until where we are today, is surely due to the long period of uncertainty of what the causes of the disease were. Long before the sugar content could be determined in the blood of an individual with (complex) technologies such as the glucometer – the technology you will come to meet more thoroughly soon – urine was the only pointer when it came to reveal disease. Urine was examined for appearance (is the urine frothy? Are there traces of blood?), color (is it dark yellow or translucent?) and taste (is it salty, bitter or perhaps sweet?) (Dods 2013: 37). Depending on the composition of the urine, the physician could draw conclusions about a possible underlying disease. In the case of diabetes, it was especially the taste of urine that made it possible to uncover the sweetness, then the sugar and therefore the disease in the first place[15]. When sugar in the urine of diabetes patients was identified as glucose in the early 19th century, this drove forth the development of early urine tests that did not merely rely on the visual appearance and the taste.

The earliest test documented is the so-called fermentation test, developed by Professor Francis Home from Edinburgh in 1780, when he detected sugar in the urine of a patient by reacting it with yeast – the first clinical technique for testing urine of diabetes patients (Schadewaldt 1989: 64). As for today, biochemists can explain that in the process of fermentation, glucose is transformed into ethanol and carbon dioxide and that "the formation of the carbon dioxide is observed as bubbles and can be used as a [...] determination of the concentration of the glucose present [...]. As the sugar content of the urine of non-diabetics is negligible, a positive fermentation test would clearly identify urine from a diabetic" (Dods 2013: 37). In the following decades urine remained the marker to uncover diabetes and the fermentation test was the gold standard for determining the existence of glucose in urine. The presence of glucose in urine was nonetheless no way of drawing conclusions about the quantity of glucose.

To prove the evidence of sugar in blood was a lot more complicated. For the first analyses of blood sugar not only enormous quantities of blood were necessary, but one analysis alone took two days in the 19th century. It was not before 1910 that one test could be performed in less than half an hour (Schadewaldt 1989: 66). In 1913, Frederick Allen, one of the leading diabetologists of his time, called out for the need to develop a clinical method that allowed an easier procedure for the quantification of blood sugar for diagnostic purposes. Though there were improvements concerning the sample volume and precision, these tests "were limited and mainly confined to diagnosis and critical care management" and still far away from being used for monitoring purposes (Clarke and Foster 2012: 84).

---

15 Tasting ones' urine in order to find out whether it tastes sweet or not is a method still used today in Uganda, though rather rarely. Though this method allows some clues on whether or not there is glucose in the urine, it cannot assist in quantifying how much glucose it is. Quantifying glucose, however, is the baseline on which medication can be adjusted and prescribed and the severity of the disease can be assessed.

The go-ahead especially for the monitoring of diabetes was reached through the development of a dry-reagent test strip for urinary glucose measurements in 1928[16]. Until 1957, the previous years of determined research and the mission to find more convenient and specific methods for glucose measurements payed off with the introduction of a "dip and read" urine reagent strip, named Clinistix (ibid.: 85). Still, this progress could not adumbrate the limitations this 'dip and read testing' entailed: the consumption of fluids as well as the concentration of the urine were influencing factors when it came to the sensitivity of the test. Furthermore, glucose in urine can only be a retrospective marker of the actual glycemic status, being inappropriate as point-of-care method. Positive results when using Clinistix will only occur when the threshold value for glucose in the kidneys is surpassed and thus may vary in cases where diabetes has been present a long time. In addition, if the strip indicates a negative result, it will not differentiate between too high sugar levels (hyperglycemia), too low sugar levels (hypoglycemia), and normal glucose levels as the correlation concerning urine and plasma glucose was revealed to be unreliable (Hayford et al. 1983: 42). Though Clinistix is still used for urinary testing today, blood became the preferred reagent for determining the presence and quantity of glucose in 'real time' (Clarke and Foster 2012: 85).

It was 1965 when the first testing strip was developed, which could use blood instead of urine: "a large drop of blood (approximately 50–100μL) was applied to the reagent pad, and after one minute the surface blood was gently washed away and the pad colour visually assessed against a colour chart to give a semiquantitative blood glucose value" (ibid.). Depending on the lighting conditions and the visual abilities of the testing person it was not always easy to visualize the correct color shades to achieve correct readings; limitations that paved the way and spurred on the motivation to develop "an automatic, electronic glucose test strip reader to improve precision and give more quantitative blood glucose results" (ibid.). The first glucometer was developed in the 1970s. A major development not only from urine to blood, but away from the laboratories to people's homes.

Glucometers are, next to the discovery of insulin, an influential invention when it comes to improving the lives of individuals with diabetes (Tonyushkina and Nichols 2009: 972). Next to the discovery of insulin, the invention of the first glucometer by Anton Clemens from the Ames Research Divisions/Miles Laboratories in Indiana, USA, using blood and not urine as reagent, can be seen as the second revolution in the (hi)story of diabetes, now more than 40 years ago. Since then, glucometers have undergone major advancements from former bulky and 1.2 kg-heavy machines (Clarke and Foster 2012: 86) kept stationary in doctors' offices, towards small, handy and easy to use point-of-care devices, intended to belong to the inventory of any diabetes patient – delivering results anywhere, fast and

---

16 Using the key enzyme glucose oxidase.

with little effort. The glucometer has an important stand as technology, "which influenced the extensive growth of point-of-care testing in the mid-1980s" (ibid.). As a diabetologist in Uganda told me "keeping this old and huge machine as a monument, will remind us of the time how it used to be."

The self-monitoring of diabetes has been essential within the treatment regime of diabetes since some decades now. A great deal of supposed simplification of self-monitoring has been brought along with the introduction of these glucometers (we will see later in this book that this is by no means always the case for everybody). This has – for some thankfully, for others regretfully – transformed into a battle between companies of who is able to design and produce the smallest and best device. The smaller, the better, the more it does not look like a medical device and is obtrusively the better. The faster it spits out a number, the better, and if it is easy to use, reliable and purchasable at an affordable price, even better. Glucometers were produced for diabetes patients in order for them to be able to test themselves at home or wherever and whenever they feel they need to do so. That they are not bound to one fixed place, meant a major breakthrough for the self-monitoring of diabetes. Therefore, you will not only be able to find them in laboratories but especially in the homes of patients who have diabetes. At least this statement holds true for individuals with diabetes in the minority world.

We will have a closer look at the glucometer and its translations as well as (self-)monitoring practices in more detail later in this book. For now, it is important to keep in mind that an individual in the minority world has the agony of choice to select a glucometer between hundreds of different models and sizes, struggling to find the glucometer that is most suitable and geared towards an individual's needs. In Uganda, it is less about choosing between an array of devices, but rather about the ability, or the chance as I will later argue in chapter five, to access them in the first place. In fact, there are only a few glucometers available on the market. While people in the minority world have the agony of choice, the majority of people in Uganda have the agony of possibility. There are simply not many possibilities to choose from. Foremost only few diabetics in Uganda are able to afford having a glucometer in their homes. While the glucometer is designed for home use, away from the laboratories to peoples' homes, in Uganda glucometers can hardly be found outside the laboratories or outside of a hospital environment. Where there was an intended movement away from the laboratories, we can observe the opposite or simultaneous movement in Uganda – back to the laboratories.

Testing matters: diagnostic tests and diagnostic criteria

There are different diagnostic tests available to diagnose diabetes. The World Health Organization together with the International Diabetes Federation (WHO and IDF

2006) have described the main three methods for diagnosis and have discussed the advantages and disadvantages of each test, which shall shortly be presented here: the OGTT, the oral glucose tolerance test; the HbA1c, glycated hemoglobin; and a blood test based on the FPG, fasting plasma glucose. What all these tests have in common is that the product of the test will be a number, which can classify an individual in three categories: non-diabetic, pre-diabetic and diabetic.

The OGTT involves dispute especially between the ADA and WHO over whether this test is an appropriate method for diagnosis or not. An individual will have to come to the test fasting, meaning without caloric intake for at least eight hours. On coming to the hospital, the person will be tested a first time. Afterwards an individual will be asked to ingest a clearly defined amount of sugar dissolved in water to be tested again afterwards and then a last time after one or two hours to see how fast and if at all the body was capable of processing the sugar. The test itself can take up to three hours. While the ADA discourages the use of this test due to the "inconvenience, greater cost and less reproducibility" (ADA 2004: 3160; see also ADA 2011), this is the recommended test by the WHO.

When I visited a private laboratory in Kampala, the laboratory technician elaborated on the OGTT the following:

> "It is a good test, but the only reason why we do it is when we are not yet sure whether someone is diabetic, they show they are beyond the normal limit. However, it is not possible for us to declare them diabetic because they are not at the upper limit. We begin to think they have an impaired glucose tolerance. The bodies are struggling to tolerate the glucose. We want to prove, is it glucose intolerance or diabetes? The issue is that most of them later graduate into diabetes if not handled. This is common with pregnant mothers. You find their sugars are unstable here and there and they are not qualified as diabetic but yet you cannot call them non-diabetic. So, we go for the test, we do the fasting glucose, then we give them an amount of glucose as powder mixed in water and then we let them take it, so we want to see after one hour how their bodies tolerate the glucose. You find for those people who have impaired glucose, it will be higher than the normal, but not necessarily in the diabetic zone [...]. The beauty about it is if they are taught how to eat, what to eat, they can reverse it. However, if they are not helped early enough they can never reverse it. Because it is a transition, it means their bodies are failing and later you will see them in the diabetic zone. It is just that many doctors do not go for it; it has a lot of psychological torture. We take off a sample three times: the patient is going to sit for three hours, sometimes even four. In those three hours they must not eat anything. They will just go for fasting glucose, [...] though it is the best test if we want to understand if it is impaired glucose tolerance. But you see, most health settings in the government area do not have what it takes because even the glucose, it may mean the patient

has to buy it, the government does not cater for that. They will say go and buy the glucose. There are many laboratory technicians who do not understand the process; they may not be able to understand how it is done."

The WHO explains that the OGTT should be the golden standard diagnostic test, because testing an individual with a fasting plasma glucose alone (as it is the case when a glucometer is applied) would not capture about 30% of undiagnosed individuals with diabetes. Moreover, this test would be, as already described by the laboratory technician above, the only means to identify individuals with the so-called IGT, impaired glucose tolerance (WHO 2006: 2).[17] In Uganda this test was, however, not applied in any of the governmental hospitals I visited. Considering the large patient numbers on a single diabetes-clinic day, this test would be too cumbersome, inconvenient and not practicable anyway (Mayega 2014).

The HbA1c is another analytic test for diabetes. HbA1c is a long-term marker, which reflects the average plasma glucose of about three months retrospectively. Unlike the OGTT and the FPG it "can be performed at any time of the day and does not require special preparation such as fasting" (WHO and IDF 2006: 32). As a laboratory technician of a private clinic in Kampala told me "[w]e go in and look for those other tests that can help us to know if this is diabetes, the HbA1c at least can give us an average of glucose of three months, it is just great. Glucose is stable in red blood cells for at least three months. So, when I have that at least it gives a better picture if this is a diabetic person. The glucometer cannot run this test. The challenge is, how many labs [laboratories] or people can afford to run this HbA1c?" While this test is suitable for already diagnosed individuals to check whether or not their glucose levels are and have been stable, the laboratory machines require regular and strict quality controls, otherwise fluctuations in the glucose levels and gray areas might occur, which make a diagnosis questionable. Furthermore, as the WHO puts it, "favourable aspects of HbA1c need to be balanced against the reality that HbA1c measurement is not widely available in many countries throughout the world" (ibid.). Additionally, anemia, which is common in under-resourced settings, may influence the results and bring about falsely diagnosed or undiagnosed

---

17 IGT, impaired glucose tolerance refers to a state in which an individual has higher glucose levels than the normal values, and lower levels than the cut-off values for being diagnosed with diabetes. This state is sometimes also referred to as 'pre-diabetes'. Nevertheless, WHO and IDF discourage using this term to avoid negative associations and stigma related to diabetes (WHO and IDF 2006: 33). The state of IGT offers the possibility of still preventing the disease by taking respective measures. However, it is important to say that I have not come across any individual who was identified as having an impaired glucose tolerance in the governmental as well as private hospitals and clinics I have visited. The field of IGT nevertheless offers an interesting field of study concerning presumptive diagnosis and diagnostic labelling in chronic disease and what this state between health and disease does to an individual.

individuals. Therefore, HbA1c is temporarily perceived as an inappropriate test for the diagnosis of diabetes. In Uganda this test is hardly available in governmental facilities. In most cases private laboratories offer this test, which then has to be paid out of one's own pocket, which is often not feasible for the diabetes patients in Uganda.

Finally, there is a blood test based on FPG, fasting plasma glucose[18]. This is the test, which we will mainly encounter in this book, as it is the principal diagnostic test performed in Uganda's governmental health facilities: An individual will be requested to come to the health center fasting. Then a drop of blood will be drawn from the fingertip and subsequently the glucose level will be determined with a glucometer. The WHO recommends using venous plasma glucose, blood from the veins, for example through a blood sample from the crook of the arm, as method for the diagnosis of diabetes; instead of using capillary blood, which is drawn from the fingertip or the lobe of the ear for instance (WHO 2006: 2). A professor specialized on diabetes diagnostics from a German university explained to me in an interview that the glucose values in capillary blood would generally be higher, for which reason venous blood would now be preferred. Whereas the results between capillary and venous blood samples may be similar in a fasting state, there is significant difference in the results in non-fasting individuals. This is why health personnel have to be certain that an individual has not eaten before the test, as the result can then easily be beyond the cut-off values and "produce" an individual with diabetes, though in fact the disease is non-existent. The WHO acknowledges the fact that instead of using venous blood for diagnosis, capillary sampling, as it is the case when a glucometer is used, is the most common practice especially in "under-resourced countries" (WHO 2006: 2). The laboratory technician in the private laboratory told me that "if you do not have these other machines, there is nothing else you can do, then you will simply use the glucometer." FPG is simpler to perform and it is not as costly as the other tests (Mayega 2014: 7).

All three tests are (in the case of Uganda it often remains theory as stated before) utilized for the diagnosis of diabetes, as well as for screening[19] practices (ADA 2016). The ADA (2016) as well as the WHO (2015) have stated the specific criteria that should be present in order to formulate a diagnosis of diabetes. I do not want to go too much into detail at this point. Yet what you are able to see and what has

---

18 In fact, all three tests (OGTT, HbA1c and FPG) are based on Plasma Glucose. But it is the FPG that utilizes the fasting state of an individual at the time of testing that differs essentially from the other tests.
19 Screening refers to the testing of individuals e.g. within a certain community "to detect diseases early in asymptomatic individuals and to treat them in order to reduce morbidity, mortality and the associated costs" (Saquib et al. 2015: 265). We will encounter screening practices in Uganda later in chapter seven, where we will have a closer look at some of the effects these practices may bring along.

been stated before: no matter which diagnostic test is applied, the product will be a number, which will then categorize a patient accordingly. How these criteria are handled in practice in Uganda, will be the matter of the next chapter. Only so much be said, it is the number that is decisive. The number reflecting the amount of sugar in the blood, sometimes together in an interplay with the typical symptoms of hyperglycemia (frequent urination, insatiable thirst, weight loss etc.). Although there is consensus between the WHO and the ADA on the diagnostic criteria for diabetes, which have evolved over time and are "based on the accumulating body of evidence" (Kumar et al. 2016: 396), there remains contestation and dispute especially over the cut-off values describing the normal lower limit of the fasting plasma glucose (ibid.). Manderson and Smith-Morris (2010) state that the

> American Diabetes Association (ADA) sets the thresholds for diabetes in ways that will capture those at great risk for later complications. That is, a diagnosis of diabetes is not so much a measurement of current problems as it is a statistically determined threshold for predicting future complications and outcomes. Screening tests to identify disease before any bodily symptoms are present offer an important advantage in biomedicine and public health [...]. Because of the importance of this diagnostic cutoff for prevention work, and because diagnostic decisions are constantly updated with new epidemiological and clinical information, the boundary line between diabetic and nondiabetic is frequently debated in the clinical literature. For many reasons that are both lay and professional diabetes is a controversial and contested diagnosis. (ibid.: 27)

Diabetes is therefore not as scientifically mastered as often perceived even in the minority world. It is and remains subject to ongoing debates, controversies and contestations on how and when a person can or should be labeled diabetic and when not.

This chapter had a threefold intention: firstly, it aimed at defining diabetes from a biomedical perspective and with this as a chronic condition. Chronic diseases are per definition characterized by their longevity and therefore can be contrasted against acute diseases where the treatment is designed towards cure and the outcome is predictable. In chronic conditions, there might be relief through appropriate treatment, but there will be no cure and the progression of the disease will remain uncertain. This has important implications for the understanding of the disease as lifelong condition on the one hand. On the other, it exerts an essential impact on aspects of care and the ability of an individual to handle and understand the disease, and how an individual may try to regain control in an uncertain life with a chronic disease.

Secondly, by outlining the short (hi)story of diabetes – transforming from a former mysterious and unknown disease to a reasonably well-understood and manageable condition – this part aimed at displaying the alleged human mastery over a disease and its transition from a deadly disease to a chronic condition brought along through technological advancements. Yet the (hi)story of diabetes as it can be found in text books and research journals, presented itself as a disease telling the story from a clearly "Western" vantage point. In Uganda, there is hardly any proof of the disease existing before the 1980s, the (hi)story of diabetes is a story and a disease that is still in the making in Uganda and other countries.

Lastly, this chapter shortly described the diagnostic tests that are available in theory today, whereby the diagnosis and the testing of diabetes in Uganda is mainly based on the use of glucometers – especially in governmental health care facilities. Therefore, pondering on the advantages and disadvantages of different diagnostic tests appears trivial if we consider that the ability of performing a diagnostic test has to be viewed against the backdrop of its access, its availability and whether or not it is feasible in the first place. The presentation of the different diagnostic tests in this chapter should not whitewash the reality that these tests are in fact often not available in a setting like Uganda. Which implications does this have for the understanding of diagnosis and testing? We will have the chance to reflect on the rationalities and realities of diagnosis in Uganda later in the empirical body of this book.

I therefore suggest that non-communicable diseases are caught in a vortex of suspense. They are provoked by the rigidity and partially the inflexibility of the regimes of global health in this 21st century, which is dedicated to global health security and humanitarian biomedicine. Though global health intends to improve the health outcomes on a global scale, it might be at the expense of conditions that do not fall in either of these two rubrics that global health dictates. As a possible result, global action is only slowly taken up, donors seemingly have little interest to engage their philanthropic endeavors and invest in this area of global health. Therefore, there is a huge lack of funding and local policies and guidelines remain stagnant. Further the lack of comprehensive numerical data is one major reason for why diabetes struggles to be seen in Uganda's health care system and beyond. Different types of evidence, such as narratives and ethnographic evidence, or "real-life evidence" as an informant once said, then become ever more important to make diabetes and the individuals who are affected by it seen.

2. (Un)measured yet (un)seen

> We used to think of it as a simple transition: from infectious diseases to a situation of non-infectious diseases, the NCDs [non-communicable diseases]. The reality of this matter is that they occur concurrently. It is a global issue. But here it used to be looked at as a dichotomy. That there were NCDs in one part of the world and we had infectious diseases in this part of the world. But now they are both here and we did not prepare in time ——Member of the Ministry of Health Uganda 2012

As early as 1989 the World Health Organization (WHO) recognized diabetes as a global health issue. Global as in it concerns all of us, and global in the sense that it can occur everywhere, in *any*-body. Even if this statement sounds fairly self-evident, it by no means is or always was. During the 42nd World Health Assembly from May 8th to May 19th in the year 1989, the WHO postulated for the first time that diabetes "already represents a significant burden on the public health services of Member States, and that the problem is *growing, especially* in developing countries" (WHA42.36, WHO 1989; my emphasis). One of the recommendations resulting from this assembly was that member states should act, *evaluate* the significance of diabetes and apply measures "appropriate to the local situation, to prevent and control diabetes" (ibid.). Two years later and in line with the WHO, King et al. (1991) published the article "Diabetes in adults is now a third world problem", appealing to the global public to start working on national health policies and interventions, which could contribute to halt the rise of diabetes. Reaching three conclusions the authors state that firstly, a diabetes "epidemic" is arising globally; secondly, that life-style and socioeconomic change are a significant factor in contributing to this epidemic; and finally, that "it is the populations in developing countries, and the minority or disadvantaged communities in the industrialized countries who now face the greatest risk [of diabetes]. [It should therefore] *now* be considered not only as a disease of industrialized countries, but *also* as a *Third World problem*" (King et al. 1991: 643; my emphasis).

Twenty-eight years have passed since the WHO held the meeting in New York recognizing and emphasizing diabetes as a global issue, and 26 years since the abovementioned article was written by King and his colleagues. Years, in which diabetes was seemingly (re)made and proclaimed a disease that was now no longer a concern only of the minority world, but also of the majority world. "A *new* disease", as I would often come to hear in Uganda. A disease on the rise, with growing numbers, reaching epidemic proportions. The previous chapter has shown that, considering the time that has passed since the discovery of a medical condition called diabetes, we can hardly speak of a new disease. Diabetes was not new – meaning no longer the mysterious and puzzling like it still had been during the lifetime of Aretaeus – when the WHO had proclaimed diabetes a global issue or when the article by King et al. was written 1991. Rather it is an old disease, framed in a new way. New "problematizations," to recall Michel Foucault's expression (1998) meaning "new ways of describing and interpreting the world – and therefore transforming it" (Fassin 2012a: 113).

Transformations take time and therefore the widely spreading claims of dramatically increasing numbers of chronic diseases, such as diabetes, seemingly cut across the actions taken to tackle them, as I intend to show in this chapter. Non-communicable diseases do not spread through viruses or bacteria transcending and ignoring national borders threatening the health of populations in the way infectious diseases do (cf. chapter three). Allen et al. (2017) argue that framing the *new* threat of the 21st century (cf. Sheridan 2012; Bygbjerg 2012; Marrero et al. 2012; Omoleke 2013; Lopez et al. 2014) as *non*-communicable diseases "propagates confusion, undermines efforts to spur a sense of urgency, and deflects attention from effective system-wide interventions [asking the challenging question whether] social injustice, globalisation, or socioeconomic transitions [may not be perceived as] causative pathogens?" (Allen et al. 2017: e129f.).[1] Chronic diseases constitute a different kind of emergency requiring a new framing and understanding of urgency as compared to infectious diseases, for they affect individuals rather than populations. They require different – long term – medical attention and care[2] (Reynolds Whyte 2014a).

In this chapter I intend to shed light on the apparent incongruity between claims of rising numbers of diabetes on the one hand and the fragmentation and supposedly lack of numerical evidence on the other, which could support these claims. There is no possibility to assess whether or not diabetes is really a new disease in countries of the majority world, or whether it has been present all along.

---

1 In their article Allen et al. (2017) question the naming of the disease group as non-communicable and call for alternatives of doing justice to the threat NCDs pose to the global public.
2 Since the establishment of the antiretroviral therapy (ART) HIV is no longer only an infectious disease, but has emerged to a chronic disease itself. Since it, however, has this dual characteristic of being infectious and chronic, I will not follow up on it in this book. Yet there are approaches that foster to think e.g. HIV/AIDS and diabetes or other chronic diseases together (cf. Janssens et al. 2007).

Therefore, instead of speaking of diabetes in terms of an old versus a new disease, or an old versus a new problem, I suggest that NCDs in general, and diabetes specifically, in Uganda and elsewhere are best understood in terms of their (in)visibility (Whyte et al. 2015) and the awareness related to it. In this way, we may better comprehend the forces that are at play in a world of the (new) global health and the world of metrics (Adams 2013) we live in today, and how claims of rising numbers might be reinforced with other forms of evidence, which are not necessarily numerical. A world in which "[w]hat gets measured gets done"– like the former director general of the WHO, Margaret Chan, once said.[3] What gets measured, however, is not only done in form of political and medical action, but it also becomes visible, expressible and tangible and with this the awareness of it increases. What is not measured, on the contrary, remains unseen, invisible and abstract in through the lens of global health and its reliance on metrics. It is then, when other forms of evidence such as anecdotes and therefore other forms of visibility may become relevant and indispensable.

Global health has become "fashionable" (Koplan et al. 2009: 1993) and is a buzzword in our world today. The attempts to define global health are numerous and it has found its way into academia, has entered the media, has been warmly welcomed by governments as an important constituent of foreign affairs and has developed into "a philanthropic target". Global health can "be thought of as a notion (the current state of global health), an objective (a world of healthy people, a condition of global health), or a mix of scholarship, research and practice (with many questions, issues, skills and competencies)" (ibid.). Evolved from its 'ancestors' colonial health and international health, global health "in the sixty-year-old postcolonial infrastructure of transnational health aid is not a simple case of new bottles for old wine. [Instead] [e]mergent trends attending to the desires for global health reveal complex transformations on the practices of audit, funding, and intervention" (Adams 2016: 1). While the previous 'health', *international* health, mainly focused on the control of epidemics between different nations, the newer term *global* health "implies consideration of the health needs of the people of the whole planet above the concerns of particular nations […]. The term 'global' is also associated with the growing importance of actors beyond governmental or intergovernmental organizations and agencies – for example, the media, internationally influential foundations, nongovernmental organizations, and transnational corporations" (Brown et al. 2006: 62).

Didier Fassin (2014) has critically engaged with the term global health and the self-evidence that seemingly comes along and adding for consideration that "beyond its overwhelming presence and apparent self-evidence, it might not be irrele-

---

3 http://www.theguardian.com/global-development/poverty-matters/2012/sep/11/non-communicable-diseases-development-goals.

vant to question whether health was less global when we did not think of it as global health. We might indeed come to wonder, how much global there can be in the local or whether a global response to diabetes for instance can function as a "magic bullet" in the sense of one size fits all, or how much local there has to be in the global? Magic bullet approaches have been the key in international health strategies and interventions for decades, "the delivery of health technologies (usually new drugs or devices) that target one specific disease without regard to the myriad societal, political, and economic factors that influence outcomes" (Biehl and Petryna 2013: 3; cf. Biehl and Petryna 2014; Clark 2014; Lorenz 2007). Adams and her colleagues (2016) have come to define global health as "*both* a response to exigencies of finance data, and outcomes that have defined the postwar world of international health and a utopian proposition to escape, if not transcend, the problems and perceived lack of success of these arrangements and exigencies" (Adams 2016: 2; emphasis in the original).

No matter how we may come to define global health or from which angle and through which lens we intend to look at it, three regimes seem to reign over the world of global health: *global health security* and *humanitarian biomedicine* (Lakoff 2010) and the strive for metrics and measurability. *Global health security* on the one hand is concerned with preventing the minority world from the threat of "emerging infectious diseases", which may be spreading from the majority world – enabled by the circulation and mobility of humans, goods, technologies and pathogens (cf. Lakoff and Collier 2008). Humanitarian biomedicine on the contrary places underserved countries at the center of attention with the "suffering individual" at its core "creating 'apolitical' networks among researchers, local health workers, private industry, and activists. At work in this regime is the notion that in order to get health care to individuals, 'intervention is seen as necessary where public health infrastructure at the nation-state level is in poor condition or non-existent' (Lakoff 2010: 61, Tichenor 2016: 107). The third regime finally, can be seen – as mentioned before – in the superelevation, strive and reliance on "specific kinds of quantitative metrics that make use of evidence-based statistical measures, experimental research platforms, and cost-effectiveness rubrics for even the most intractable health problems and most promising interventions" (Adams 2016: 1; we will dig deeper into this in the following conceptual chapter of this book).

Diabetes falls in neither of the first two regimes as described by Lakoff really (2010); it does not spread from the majority world to the minority world[4] threatening its health security, and it has it so far not attracted many humanitarian efforts and or great support (we will have a look at this aspect of global health in more detail in chapter seven). The strive for numbers in the case of NCDs in the majority

---

4 In fact, the opposite could be the case for it was a disease, and the idea of this disease, which spread from the minority world to the majority world.

world also seems to lag behind. I propose to frame diabetes as a disease caught up in a vortex of suspense induced by the rigidity and partially inflexibility of the *new* global health in the 21st century. Narayan et al. (2013) stress the importance of good surveillance systems for non-communicable diseases, which

> are crucial for measuring the magnitude of the problem and its associated costs, identifying vulnerable sub-groups, and evaluating the effects of policy and practice interventions, especially in low- and middle-income countries where such data are woefully lacking. Serious global commitments to basic and applied research are essential; research is currently overwhelmingly concentrated in high-income countries, but the burden of non[-]communicable diseases is felt around the globe. (Narayan et al. 2013: 876)

It is a vortex of suspense fed by lacking numerical evidence, deficient financial aid and medical interventions and the discrepancy between awareness and responsiveness.

Number business

Good health is understood not only as a fundamental to human well-being but also as sine qua non for progress and change and has emerged to an essential component of any global development planning agenda (Dave 2016: 85; Biehl and Petryna 2013). For the United Nations Millennium Summit in September of the year 2000, in the wake of a new millennium, 147 heads of state were mobilized to assemble at the United Nations Headquarters in New York "to shape a broad vision to fight poverty in its many dimensions [and to] spare no effort to free our fellow men, women and children from the abject and dehumanizing conditions of extreme poverty [...] and [to] address the health needs that arise from the scourge of infectious diseases" (UN, The Millennium Development Goals Report 2015: 3). The outcome of this meeting culminated in the formulation of the so-called Millennium Development Goals (MDGs): compiled into eight key goals the aim was to create an all-encompassing framework and agenda for development for a timeframe of 15 years. The MDGs became a keyword and an important tool in global health, which could not be bypassed when working with issues related to development in any of its multiple facets. Three of the eight goals, goal four, five and six, were directly linked to health (goal 4: Reduce Child Mortality; goal 5: Improve Maternal Health; and goal 6: Combat HIV/AIDS, malaria and other diseases)[5] (ibid.: 5f): the Millennium Declaration fostered to reduce the maternal mortality by three

---
5 The full list of MDGs can be found on http://www.un.org/millenniumgoals/ (last accessed 24th of March 2017).

quarters, to decrease the under-five mortality by two-thirds and to halt and reverse the spread of HIV, malaria and "other major diseases that afflict humanity" (UN Millennium Declaration, 8th of September 2000). At the close of the 15 years, in 2015, the United Nations published a report displaying the achievements and promoted the MDGs as "the most successful anti-poverty movement in history" (ibid.; see also UN 2011; 2007). Enriched with a large quantity of metrics, including numbers, tables and charts, the MDGs, was stated, would prove "that, with targeted interventions, sound strategies, adequate resources and political will, even the poorest countries can make dramatic and unprecedented progress" (ibid.).

What the report omitted to document was that despite the recorded progress, many countries were in fact still far off to reach the MDGs. As Easterly (2008) states, the MDGs "were meant as a major motivational device to increase development efforts in and on behalf of poor countries, and the resulting publicity and aid increases suggest they can claim considerable achievement on that score" (ibid.: 26). Yet the MDGs were not only a tool for improvement or an anti-poverty movement, but instead they created a basis on which the achievements but also the failures of a country could be assessed, evaluated and measured. On a number of occasions, especially Sub-Saharan Africa has been compared to other more "successful" countries and its underperformance has been highlighted. It seemed to be unquestionable that Sub-Saharan Africa would not reach the eight goals. Quotes such as: "At the midway point between their adoption in 2000 and the 2015 target date for achieving the MDGs, Sub-Saharan Africa is not on track to achieve any of the Goals" (United Nations 2007) or "[…] at the mid point of the MDGs, Sub-Saharan Africa is the only region which, at current rates, will meet none of the MDG targets by 2015" (Africa Progress Panel 2007, Easterly 2008: 27) – statements representing a judgmental flavor of the MDGs. Considering that most of the targets were "implausible" for many countries in the first place, Clemens et al. highlight the "rapid progress by historical standards" the countries underwent nevertheless (Clemens et al. 2007: 735; see also Andrews et al. 2015).

While focusing on countries in Sub-Saharan Africa (among others) and how well they were performing – expressed through numbers – what was despite all the shortcomings called "the most successful anti-poverty movement in history", obscured the pitfalls and excluding mechanisms that came along as well. The formulation of the MDGs as well as the report at the end of the MDG-era display one thing quite clearly: unlike HIV/AIDS and malaria, subsumed under goal number six and clearly designated to "combat HIV/AIDS, malaria and other major diseases", non-communicable diseases were not included explicitly.[6] They were invisible in

---

6 Indeed, other diseases were not mentioned explicitly either. But given the fact, that NCDs are said to be the main killer globally, it does give reason to ask why they have not been stated

the list of MDGs and remained invisible in the reports. Yet as Adams (2016) insinuates "doing global health [today] means caring an awful lot about numbers. Being able to count what it is we are doing seems to matter more than ever before [...]. The Millennium Development Goals might be hard to reach, but it is not hard to see that the only way to know if we have reached them is if we have good ways of measuring the outcomes of what we are doing now" (ibid.: 23). Accomplishments of HIV and malaria interventions, conditions for which there were numbers, were highlighted at the expense of other diseases, such as NCDs, though they had already been understood as a global threat when the MDGs were formulated. According to Oni-Orisan (2016) the increasing reliance on numbers is problematic for if they start "circulating in this political way, it becomes difficult to question them [and] [t]heir power multiplies" (ibid.: 89). The generating of numbers and their aggrandizement do not only make a problem visible through numbers, but at the same time gains impetus and visibility, overshadowing problems and medical conditions that are looming in the dark, unmeasured and often invisible or not as visible. Accordingly, the MDGs may be seen as more than well-intentioned goals leading to positive change. They can be perceived as a device with which the performance of a country could be calculated and measured, assessed with clearly defined targets while at the same time they functioned as a device casting a cloud to make the increasing numbers of NCDs visible by omitting them in the agenda.

Goal number six of the MDGs was clearly designated to "combat HIV/AIDS, malaria and other major diseases". Despite also mentioning tuberculosis, no other disease was further considered. Was it not diabetes and other NCDs, which were at that point "major diseases" as well? In her article "Global Health Business: The Production and Performativity of Statistics in Sierra Leone and Germany", Susan Erikson (2012) highlights that the

> global push for health statistics and electronic digital health information systems is about more than tracking health incidence and prevalence. It is also experienced on the ground as means to develop and maintain particular norms of health business, knowledge, and decision- and profit-making that are not innocent. Statistics make possible audit and accountability logics that undergird the management of health at a distance and that are increasingly necessary to the business of health. Health statistics are inextricable from their social milieus, yet as business artifacts they operate as if they are freely formed, objectively originated, and accurate. (Erikson 2012: 367)

Shifting global health to a "business" has further demanded to find new ways of collecting even more numbers (ibid.: 368). Where there are no numbers, there is a

---

explicitly. In fact, when reading the report, I did not find any mentioning of diabetes specifically at all in the entire document, nor of NCDs in general.

lack of funding. Not including NCDs in the MDGs has been preventing countries from receiving donor funding as (bilateral) aid agencies would "exclusively fund the health priorities contained within the MDGs despite the fact that NCDs cause 14 million annual deaths under the age of 60 in LMICs [low- and middle-income countries]".[7] As a member in the Ministry of Health of Uganda once told me, numbers and data accelerate the pouring of resources because (international) donors as well as the government would not be interested in putting a lot of efforts in fighting a condition, which is 'non'-existent (or *non*-communicable?) or hardly visible. Biehl and Petryna (2013) state that along with the new global health there are

> a multiplicity of actors, all vying for resources and influence in the political field of global health, each seeking to remain relevant and powerful players. Ranging from the Gates Foundation to pharmaceutical company drug donation programs and PEPFAR (the [US] President's Emergency Plan for AIDS Relief), [...] these diverse interests are setting new norms for institutional response, sometimes providing the public health resources that states and markets cannot or have failed to furnish. (Biehl and Petryna 2013: 6)

It is this circumstance that has persuaded others to call diabetes the "real neglected tropical disease"[8] (Hsu and Potter 2015; Reynolds Whyte 2014a) in spite of the fact, that the World Health Organization has called the world leaders to develop national non-communicable disease (NCD) responses several times in the past already. Tichenor (2016) states that malaria for instance has been a central disease within research and development efforts in the past decades, obtaining the highest quantity of donor funds allocated to global health (next to HIV/AIDS and tuberculosis, which together form the Big Three). She relates this to the inclusion of malaria into the agenda of the MDGs after which "the number of projects and funding for combating the disease at least quadrupled in the past two decades" (ibid.: 107). NCDs are increasing and account for a significant burden of disease globally, the (financial) attention they have been receiving, however, is nominal and not matching the voices that can be heard all over the globe calling for action. The Institute for Health Metrics and Evaluation (IHME) from the University of Washington stated in their report in 2013 that NCDs received little funding in relation to their share in the burden of disease and especially when compared to communicable diseases. The development assistance for health (DAH) for HIV/AIDS for example was twenty-

---

7 https://ncdalliance.org/ncds-and-the-millennium-development-goals (accessed: 24th March 2017).
8 Neglected tropical diseases (NTDs) account for a disease group of communicable diseases, which occur in tropical and sub-tropical territories. Those living in extreme poverty without access to proper sanitation are at greatest risk of contracting an NTD. Examples for NTDs are: Dengue, Schistosomiasis and Leprosy. (WHO 2017; for the full list of NTDs visit: http://www.who.int/neglected_diseases/diseases/en/).

fold higher than the spending allocated to all NCDs together in 2011 (Dieleman and Murray, IHME 2013: 29).[9] As the NCD Alliance states on their homepage that "while the HLM [high-level meeting] Political Declaration recognised that resources are not 'commensurate with the problem' and encourages governments to explore bilateral and multilateral channels, we are yet to see a major shift in resources."

In 2011, four years left to reach the goals set by the MDGs, the UN had a high-level meeting in New York from the 19th to the 20th of September. In this meeting, global leaders stressed that the health of the global public is the inevitable requirement for development and that "success in global health cannot be achieved without bold coordinated efforts to incorporate NCDs prevention, control and care into the current workstream" (UN high level meeting New York 2011). Since the MDGs did not capture NCDs explicitly, and fueled by an increasing pressure to act (e.g. from the NCD Alliance), the UN adjusted the MDGs retroactively (11 years later) adding possible connections between the eight MDGs and NCDs (WHO 2011). Though not formally established, what was not explicitly formulated and visible in the MDGs before, was constructed afterwards: "Poverty and Hunger" for instance could be associated with NCDs because "illness, disabilities and death from NCDs hurt economic productivity and household income" (ibid.). Connecting NCDs to the MDGs afterwards could be seen as an attempt to eliminate the possibility of seeing actions taken, or rather the non-action, as a failure to take responsibility and be held accountable. There is an irony here: the same organizations that had proclaimed NCDs as a major threat were now struggling to justify their non-mentioning of NCDs and the absent actions taken.[10]

The NCD alliance, a network "uniting 2.000 civil society organisations in more than 170 countries"[11], founded in 2009, has been and continues to be one of the greatest advocates fighting for the promotion and recognition of NCDs. It was therefore perceived as a major success and step forward in the battle against NCDs when the 2030 agenda for sustainable development, entitled "Transforming our world", has formulated the so-called Sustainable Development Goals (SDGs). It has committed itself to "stimulate action over the next 15 years in areas of critical importance for humanity and the planet [while the] new Agenda builds on the Millennium Development Goals. Further it seeks to complete what they did not achieve, particularly in reaching the most vulnerable" (UN 2015a: 1). Compared to the MDGs, the number of goals has more than doubled with now 17 goals. For us interesting is especially goal number three "[e]nsure healthy lives and promote well-

---

9 In 2011 $377 million was allocated for NCDs (1.2% of the total Development Assistance for Health) of which $68 million were flown to tobacco-related programs (Dieleman and Murray, IHME 2013: 10).
10 No need to mention that the participating countries were of course working to reach the MDGs rather than focus on a group of conditions for which there is no financial support.
11 https://ncdalliance.org/.

being for all at all ages"[12], which in turn involves target number three "By 2030, reduce by one-third premature mortality from non-communicable diseases through prevention and treatment and promote mental health and well-being." These new developments meant a major breakthrough for the ongoing efforts of for instance the NCD Alliance, who stated:

> "Today is a historic moment for the non-communicable disease (NCD) community. This morning, world leaders formally adopted the 2030 *Agenda for Sustainable Development* at the **United Nations** in New York [...]. *The adoption of Agenda 2030 today marks a momentous achievement for the NCD community. It is a time when we can be more optimistic about the future of prevention and control of NCDs than perhaps at any stage of recent history.* For the first time, NCDs are included in these goals as a sustainable development priority for all countries".

These words by Ms. Katie Dain, the Executive Director of the NCD Alliance[13], are a statement full of relief, joy and hope, and reflects a moment of victory after having been fighting for the recognition of NCDs and the inclusion in the global development agenda since its establishment. Whereas the MDGs were preoccupied with eliminating poverty, hunger and infectious diseases, non-communicable diseases have now been explicitly mentioned in the Sustainable Development Goals (SDGs) (Hawkes and Popkin 2015: 1).

Though NCDs have been included in the SDGs, there was dispute around the depth and extent to which they had been included. The recognition of NCDs, according to some voices, had not led to an adequate translation of NCDs, and a definitive strategy for fighting NCDs would still be lacking (cf. Buse and Hawkes 2015; Brolan et al. 2015). Dave (2016) comments that compared to the encumbrance evoked by the global increase of NCDs, they would not be addressed sufficiently in the SDGs "therefore undermining current and future health needs. Their positioning is weak and fails to address major risk factors [...]. Arguably, in the absence of broad legal and environmental interventions, the burden of preventing and managing NCDs will fall on individuals' personal behavior changes" (ibid.: 92f.).

There is agreement that the actions taken to tackle NCDs are few, and the mills of action are grinding slower than the appreciation of the situation would require. The availability of country specific metrics on and for NCDs, without which the real burden of NCDs cannot be assessed and visualized, and with which policies could be informed and numbers could circulate and multiply their power (Oni-Orisan 2016), remains fragmented. What all reports and goals have not been mentioning

---

12 A complete list of the sustainable development goals can be found under https://sustainabledevelopment.un.org/?menu=1300.
13 The quote derives from the webpage of Union internationale contre le cancer (UICC), one of the members of the NCD Alliance: http://www.uicc.org/.

while talking about prevention and control, is the estimated number of unknown cases due to firstly a lack of diagnostic possibilities and in turn the lack of metrics, numerical evidence. Without efforts to make the (un)known visible in the case of NCDs especially in the majority world, there may be further development agendas following, without numerical evidence the struggle will continue and gain momentum very slowly.

Data in transit? A status quo of NCDs in Uganda

As pointed out before, numerical evidence is not only a driving force to inform (political) action, but also a means to make the invisible visible and quantifiable. "Not documented is not done", as health workers in Uganda tend to say. Or "What gets measured, gets done", according to the former director general of the WHO, Margaret Chan. Lacking policies and guidelines are one big issue that have led to the neglect of these diseases not only globally, but also in Uganda's health care system. Policies and guidelines are strategies to facilitate action, but also to uncover, prevent, manage and treat diseases in a formally organized and officially recognized way. The NCD surveillance system in Uganda is weak, the little data that is available is not only patchy and "very localized, and variable both in quality and methods [but] NCD data is often not sufficiently integrated into [the] national health information system while health facility records are grossly incomplete due to under-diagnosis" (Mayega 2014: 2). This chapter aims at staging NCDs at the midway of stagnant policies and commencing action, while waiting for numbers. What is done in relation to NCDs in Uganda, what are interferences in taking up action and where is Uganda heading?

One of the first things that was brought up when I visited the Ministry of Health in Uganda was the HMIS, the Health Monitoring Information System, a tool developed to enhance the outcomes of the Health Sector Strategic Plan (HSSP)[14] in 2000. "When data was generated before, it was very fragmented, inaccurate or came delayed. The capturing of data used to be haphazard", I was told. The HMIS is a tool, which intends to avoid this by enabling the collection of health-related data in a systematic way. The numbers that are generated are ultimately transmitted to the Ministry of Health of Uganda. It

> is an integrated reporting system used by the Ministry of Health, Development Partners and Stakeholders to collect relevant and functional information on a routine basis [...] to enable planning, decision making, monitoring and evaluation

---

14 The HSSP is a major component and important basis for the overall health sector planning framework in Uganda and stipulates the focus of the health care sector for a given timeframe (MoH 2015: 19).

of the health care delivery system. It is designed to assist managers carry out evidence based decision making at all levels of the health care delivery [and to] plan and coordinate health care services. (MoH, HMIS 2014: XV)

Accordingly, the HMIS can be seen as a driving force when it comes to the making of evidence, the generating of numbers and making a disease visible (e.g. on paper and then in action) and forms the baseline for all measures taken in relation to a disease. Its "relevance" in turn is, as we have seen before, nurtured not only by local, but also global perceptions of what is relevant.

Most health facilities, especially at the lower health centers (HC II and III) use the HMIS tool in a paper format. The most common health conditions are listed in a table and the recorded cases can be completed.[15] The paper forms are completed on a weekly basis, by health care workers themselves on a lower health care level and by designated data managers at the higher levels. Subsequently they are handed over to the data officer of each district headquarter who in turn is responsible for gleaning the health information from all health units in the district and digitize the information via a computerized system monthly. After the data has been collected it is handed over to the DHO, the district health officer, who is responsible for transmitting it electronically to the Ministry of Health of Uganda. Once received, the data of the whole country is gathered, stored and administered at the data resource center in Kampala. There is no regular publishing of the collected data, but if specific data for instance in form of reports on the status quo is needed for a certain disease, the resource center can be contacted and the needed data delivered – if it is available. As Dr. A. explains "if the ministry is for example making a health sector strategic plan, they know they can go there [to the resource center] and say, please, give us an idea about the malaria cases. To see the statistics in a district and to see whether over time there have been any changes, increases or decreases or whatever. There you just get general statistics." However, the diseases captured in the HMIS framework used to picture especially chronic conditions in a way, which led to confusion and therefore to a non-recording of these cases. "This is one of the reasons for a lack of numbers", Dr. A., a former employee at the Ministry of Health of Uganda, explained. "It was the complexity of the former HMIS", namely that the HMIS was not singling out the NCDs into the single diseases.

It was in 2013 when the NCD working group from the Ministry of Health was "taking up the fight against NCDs". When they held their first meeting in Kampala, they were enthusiastic and eager to "push things forward", until they realized they did not have any information about non-communicable diseases in Uganda to base their efforts on. "We knew that NCDs were out there, that they were a problem. But we did not know how serious it was, we did not have numbers. NCDs were not yet

---

15 Most health centers have additional recording books and enter the HMIS on a weekly basis.

recognized as a big problem because there was no data", one of the former project members explained. The data that was there was fragmented. After pursuing some small investigations on this matter, they realized that the health facilities were not recording any of the non-communicable diseases, because the Health Management Information System (HMIS) did not capture these conditions, or rather captured them in a way that complicated the documentation of each disease and therefore the generating of numbers. Cardiovascular diseases were listed with the abbreviation CVD, yet the overarching term was not sub-divided into the particular diseases like hypertension, heart attack or stroke. The same applied to metabolic disorders, the term under which diabetes would be categorized. Since the diseases were not singled out, and because many health workers had hard times to understand and make sense of the abbreviation "CVD" or the expression "metabolic disorders", the number in these columns remained zero and subsequently no cases of this disease-group were captured.

A measure to counteract fragmented documentation was the revision of the outdated HMIS form and NCDs, enumerated in their different components, were included into the documentation system. A process that started in the end of 2013 and lasted until August 2015, when the rollout of these new forms was driven forth. Dr. A. explained "there are so many NCDs, but I felt if we could at least get some information regularly from the health facilities, it would be useful for us, especially because then we did not even have the national survey yet. So at least going forward, we can get some information from the health units." The national prevalence for NCDs in Uganda remained unknown, had it not yet been assessed through the Uganda Demographic and Health Survey (UDHS) like other diseases, which had for so long been on the list. When I visited the Statistic Centre in Kampala for the first time in 2012, I came across a folder that had assembled all the Demographic Health Surveys that had been conducted in Uganda so far. At a first glance of the most recent surveys at that point, 2006 and 2011, I could see that NCDs had not been included in any of them. Instead the focus was on child and maternal health, family planning, vaccination and especially HIV/AIDS (UBOS 2014; 2011; 2006).[16] As is stated in the most recent Key Indicators Report of Uganda's Demographic and Health Survey:

> The main purpose of the 2016 UDHS is to provide the data needed to monitor and evaluate population, health, and nutrition programmes on a regular basis. Increasing emphasis by planners and policy makers on the utilisation of objective indicators for policy formulation, planning, and measuring progress has increased the reliance on regular household survey data, given the inadequate

---

16 So far there have been six Uganda Demographic and Health Surveys: 1988/89; 1995; 2000/01; 2006; 2011 and 2016.

availability of appropriate information from administrative statistics and other routine data-collection systems. ('Uganda Demographic and Health Survey 2016', published 2017: ix)

NCDs, again, were not included and what is referred in the report as "inadequate availability of appropriate information from administrative statistics and other routine data-collection systems" remained the only source of data for NCDs.

In 2014, a "Non-Communicable Disease Risk Factor Baseline Survey" was conducted, the first survey exclusively on NCDs. The 'STEPwise approach to surveillance' (STEPS), a tool developed and endorsed by the WHO, should support especially "low- and middle-income countries to get started in NCD prevention and control activities [with] a simplified approach providing standardized materials and methods as part of a technical collaboration with countries, especially those that lack resources" (WHO 2003: V). Based on a five-months research study, the survey sought to assess the national prevalence of diabetes and shed light on possible risk factors related to NCDs (MoH 2014a). Nearly 4000 individuals participated in the study from nine districts and the four different regions in Uganda (Central, Northern, Western and Eastern region). One of the outcomes of the survey was the Ugandan prevalence rate for diabetes of 2% among adults above the age of 18 (Bahendeka et al. 2016)[17], highlighting that the 89% of the participants were neither on medication nor had they known that they were having raised blood sugar levels (MoH 2014a).

And yet the STEPS survey was not the only action taken on NCDs in Uganda, though, as stated in a report by the Ministry of Health of Uganda, "[l]ooking at NCDs, there were limited interventions introduced to halt the rising burden of this disease group" (MoH 2015: 33). In 2008, the Danish World Diabetes Foundation (WDF) secured funds over one million US Dollars to initiate a diabetes program in Uganda. However, as Dr. A. from the Ministry of Health stated "not much was done, so they suspended the project because of non-performance." You have milestones, which you have to reach in order for the money to be provided. But the person responsible for the project at that time "did not do his work properly". The project was frozen. A few years later a team of four individuals decided to ask the WDF to take up the project again. "Because nobody was really interested in NCDs this project was so important for us", a former member of the project explained. As far as he knew, the WDF was the only donor funded project at least for diabetes in Uganda.[18]

---

17 Compared to a global diabetes prevalence of 8.5% in 2014 (WHO 2017a).
18 I encountered another project running in Uganda on diabetes, specifically targeting children with type-1 diabetes by the Danish pharmaceutical company Novo Nordisk "Changing Diabetes in Children". More information on this project can be found under: https://www.novonordisk.com/sustainability/actions/Access-to-care/CDiC.html; see also chapter six of this book.

One of the first steps of the NCD working group was to conduct a needs-assessment on NCDs by selecting a number of health facilities countrywide. 13 regions in Uganda were involved in the project and three people of each region (a doctor, a nurse and a clinical medical officer respectively) were meant to be educated and trained on NCDs. 54 Health Centers were selected of which 13 were regional referral hospitals, 27 district hospitals and 14 Health Center IVs. Each of the regional referral hospitals were supposed to be equipped with machines in order to measure the HbA1C [long-term blood sugar levels, cf. chapter one] but the procurement of these machines alone took two years. This needs-assessment sought to answer questions such as whether the health centers were offering any services for NCDs in general or not; how well they were staffed and how knowledgeable the staff was on NCDs; which equipment was available in the laboratories and if it was still functioning. They went to the dispensaries of each facility to evaluate the availability of pharmaceuticals for the treatment of individuals. The needs assessment was supposed to function as the springboard for developing a strategic plan and develop polices for NCDs. Dr. A. explained:

> "We wanted to collect some small information in order to develop a comprehensive policy and a strategic plan for our country. We realized when we had an initial meeting, called stakeholders avenue, if we documented the NCDs, at least we know they are there. But over time we needed more information to enrich the strategic plan. Since we didn't have it, we kind of shelved the policy because you cannot say, let us wait for the survey, let us wait for some kind of data to come in. We have a draft for the NCD strategic plan, draft policy, draft screening guidelines. Because we say, yes, we know there is a big problem and right now as we wait for technology, drugs and equipment, the health workers can at least pick up a few individuals and refer them early if they know what to do with an individual who is suspect of NCD. It is a challenge, because the policies stay on the table. To put out a policy needs trained people. There is no point to put out a policy if you cannot train people about it. It doesn't make sense to develop policies if the ministry doesn't have any funds, then it will stay in the shelves. Until a development partner comes and says you know what guys, we need to train everybody about diabetes or whatever. When you roll out a policy, it involves guidelines, training and what. People have to go around and train people. For the treatment of malaria for instance, we were using chloroquine or fansidar before [both medications to treat malaria] and then they changed to ACTs [artemisinin-based combination therapies]. Now this change alone must be organized somewhere in a policy and it has to be trained across the whole country. Otherwise it becomes unethical."

The lacking policies and guidelines contributed to the lack of a common message related to the management of diabetes on an individual as well as on a health center-based level. Though the needs-assessment did lead to the development of a number of guidelines for screening as well as policies they are until today in draft form, "stagnant, lying in the shelf", waiting to be implemented, when I was in Uganda the last time in October 2016. Yet all the efforts and all the blood, sweat and tears Dr. A. and her colleagues invested in bringing NCDs higher up on the agenda, were disappointed precipitously. The guidelines for screening and management of NCDs were seen as too bulky and she soon got the feeling that "the politicians only seem to do something if it is expected somehow, but it seems the project from the WDF was doomed to fail from the start". The email account of one of the project members was hacked and emails were sent to WDF via this account asking for a money transfer to a dubious bank account in Kazakhstan – since then, the project is again on hold. "Since the project was frozen, I am not getting a salary anymore and now I am thinking of stopping in this field [of NCDs], perhaps switch to malaria or HIV where there is money. I love NCDs, but I do not know where to take myself."

(Un)measured but seen – diabetes in Uganda

The more tests a glucometer will perform, the more positive cases of diabetes might be brought to light (and it appears that this is actually the case) and even more than that, for they produce more than *a* single number. Or say, this one number may function in different ways and for different purposes: one indicates the level of glucose[19], but this same number may (re-)create a patient if the glucose levels surpass the normal glucose values. This may then contribute to the collection of epidemiological data, to the making of another diabetes case. In order for this number, this patient, to count as evidence, these numbers have to be noted down, formalized and then reported. Otherwise all these numbers and perhaps (new) 'cases' of diabetes patients, the glucometer produces, remain empty, unseen and therefore useless. For them to count, they have to be made viable systematically, visible and accessible to a broader audience of local and global actors. These numbers and metrics produced on a local scale have to be *made global* in order to be able to count locally – this is what the previous chapters have revealed. It is not only the unavailability of glucometers, which may hamper the collection of data. It is the interplay between diagnostic opportunities, appropriate policies and frameworks that make eventual data useful alongside a functioning reporting system that can entrench these numbers in an infrastructural landscape and transform mere diabetes cases into valuable and actionable evidence – all these factors contribute to the making

---

19 In chapter six we will see that in the case of glucose measuring and monitoring that a number can take on the function of a placeholder or entry point between the body and the self.

of a disease. Evidence is nothing that can stand-alone; it is nothing that exists in its own right, but evidence requests for action, for response, it cries out for movement and it has no respect for latecomers. At the same time (numerical) evidence also legitimizes action and prioritizes aspects that *are* evident over the ones that might be evident, yet without the support of numbers. Or, as Daniel Neyland put it, to have "an 'evidence base' from which to proceed has become a defining logic for action" (Neyland 2013: 219).

"We did not get serious about diabetes", I hear her saying, while she seems to look into a devastating emptiness. "You know", the woman I met formerly working for the Ministry of Health of Uganda explained

> "HIV has been a big problem from some time back. Of course, it still is. But what I want to say is that everyone knows how to diagnose HIV, even malaria, but not these NCDs. From every report in every health unit, even as far down as in the village, they are able to say we have 20 malaria cases, 20 this, 20 this. But it is a different picture for diabetes [...]. Because you know when HIV came with all the global attention, there was reporting of numbers. That is why I think malaria, tuberculosis and HIV received a lot of attention because they had numbers from the beginning. There was a pouring of resources and the global players still want these same diseases. Maybe they are waiting for one of them to get knocked down by diabetes to be able to feel it themselves how big of a threat it really is. There are no efforts. Diabetes is simply not on the global agenda, because if so, people would start working on them. We realized it is a big issue in our country and it is not yet recognized as a big issue, because there was no data."

The vortex of suspense displayed in the introduction of this chapter – nurtured by a lack of numerical evidence, deficient financial aid and medical interventions alongside the divergence between awareness and responsiveness to disease – is clearly not only visible on a global level, but becomes especially visible in a local setting like Uganda. As mentioned before, the process of incorporating NCDs, and therefore diabetes, into the formal health care system of Uganda is still in its infant stage. Policies, though formulated, are remaining non-implemented, lying in the shelves of the Ministries. The landscape of NCD policies remains vague and fragmented. Numbers, scientific proof, or epidemiological data to be precise, do not only have the power to inform or facilitate actions, but they can also be used – or rather the neglect to collect numbers (cases of diabetes patients or data on NCDs in general for this matter) – to prevent or exclude from action and to make diabetes visible through the lens of global health. Yet we may come to wonder how then diabetes becomes visible and how the awareness of this disease can increase despite this alleged lack of numerical evidence? By focusing too much on the global in global health, we may come to oversee that there are indeed local explanations not only for why the numbers of diabetes are increasing but *that* they are increasing. This will be the core of this chapter. How do we come to know that something is there, if the numbers want to convince us of the contrary?

We may also ask the question whether it is really evidence, which is lacking? Whereas I remember vividly that when I was collecting data in Uganda for my Master thesis in 2012 it happened more than once that people I met had never heard of diabetes before, the situation seemed to have changed. Coming back in 2015 everybody appeared to know or at least have heard about this disease, the disease that is called "sukali", the "sugar disease", the "evil disease that kills". The evidence is there, but it is a different kind of evidence added to the fragments of numbers existing in Uganda. It is not only numerical in nature, but also anecdotal. I aim to display anecdotal evidence, or rather evidence conveyed through narratives and observations, as a tool for substituting for a lack of numerical evidence. By describing a few channels through which the rise of diabetes is conveyed in narratives, reports, observations and conversations that contribute to the *making* of diabetes in Uganda. Or as Annemarie Mol would perhaps phrase it, how diabetes is *done* in Uganda (Mol 2002: 6). Biehl and Petryna (2014) make clear that as

> ethnographers, we are uniquely positioned to see what more categorically minded experts may overlook: namely, the empirical evidence that emerges when people express their most pressing and ordinary concerns, which then open up to complex human stories in time and space and that must become the center of public reflection and action. (ibid.: 378)

One way of knowing that the cases of diabetes are rising in Uganda, is by *seeing* and *hearing* the numbers of patients growing in the health centers. As stated before, we cannot fully know what really is increasing; whether it is the numbers of cases or the awareness of this disease. Or might the increasing numbers be related to improved diagnostic possibilities and the awareness that diabetes is exactly not a disease, which only occurs in wealthier countries, but everywhere, leading individuals to seek care and consultation? Or a combination of all factors? Health care workers on the one hand described the dramatic increase in workload, because there is a true "stampede of new diabetes people in the facility." Especially individuals who were living with diabetes for a long time already were able to contrast the status quo in the health facilities today with the times when they had just been diagnosed with diabetes. "It is the people we see in the clinic, they are now too many people with diabetes. Before, I did not have to wait all day to see the doctor, but now it might take me one whole day waiting because it is only one diabetes-doctor for all these people." While the numbers of patients with diabetes were few before, health centers were now overcrowded and it was not uncommon that patients came early in the morning lining up, only to leave the health center in the late afternoon or early evening. It happened so many times that I literally had to climb over waiting people, jammed and squeezed together in the narrow hallway, in order to get to the consultation room. Especially health workers working in health facilities that offer specialized diabetes clinics reported that they could witness the increase of diabetes. A nurse working in a specialized diabetes clinic of a governmental health facility said "every time there is a clinic day, I register new patients." While opening the big blue NCD registration book, she said, "see, these ones are new, those ones are new. These are new and this one was the worst one today, with life threatening glucose levels."

The NCD registration books have been introduced by the Medical Research Council of Uganda (MRC), a research unit, usually preoccupied with research related to HIV. However, they have conducted a pilot project on NCDs in a selected number of governmental health facilities in different districts of Uganda (predominantly diabetes and hypertension). A specialized documenting system was initiated through the provision of NCD registration books (which is common practice for HIV in Uganda) as well as supplying diagnostic equipment and medication detached from the usual governmental supply system through the National Medical Stores (NMS).[20] This on the one hand led to a situation of rather well-equipped diabetes clinics, barely any stock outs of medication or testing equipment. But on the other to an even greater increase of patients in these supported facilities after it had gotten around among health workers and patients that the services in these facilities were a lot better as compared to other governmental health centers, which were not part of the research program. Against the backdrop of this improved infrastructure for diabetes care, the MRC started to encourage these health centers to extend their usual practice not only to test, when an individual shows the typical symptoms, but to engage in screening practices as well. Meaning that every individual who fulfills certain criteria will automatically be tested for diabetes even though she might not have any complaints or symptoms. Like a health worker explained "[w]e screen every day. Any patient who is 18 years and above will be screened for hypertension, that is we check for high blood pressure. Then for diabetes, we use our four F's: anyone who is **F**orty years, who is **F**at, who **F**requently urinates and who has diabetes in the **F**amily. If someone matches all four F's, we test". This in turn has created overly crowed health facilities and due to the rise of patients, again to a limited availability of medicines and medical equipment.[21] A patient told me that

> "they chased us away from Mulago hospital [the national referral hospital of Uganda]. So, we decided to come this side [to this health facility]. This led to a scarcity of medicine. It is a very big problem because the medicine is no longer enough for us. The doctors try hard to see that each and everyone gets medicine,

---

20 Unfortunately, I cannot go into detail on the research project by MRC. Attempts to get in touch with them were left unanswered.
21 We will frequently encounter this issue in the empirical chapters of this book.

but still it cannot be enough. Some have resorted to buying medicine from the private pharmacies and other private hospitals, which is costly. Even when it comes to testing, the strips are not enough. There are simply too many of us."

What comes along with *seeing* increased numbers is that all actors involved *feel* the increased numbers. Especially the patients will feel that due to the high number of patients, the resources are limited and not enough for everybody. The health workers feel the increased numbers, because they will have to work late hours, often not even able to take a ten minutes' break.

A diabetologist I met, Dr. E., told me that partly the increasing numbers are related to the growing awareness and knowledge about diabetes. Before, there was not the knowledge about these conditions and the diagnostic possibilities to reveal the disease in the first place were limited. An individual would have just died without knowing it was diabetes that killed. "People used to die, but they did not know they were dying of diabetes. So, people used to pass on and some thought they were bewitched" a patient mentioned. But now, since the numbers were increasing, and awareness was increasing, the knowledge of this disease was also increasing.

In medical schools in Uganda, diabetes was not taught much either. It was taught a little, but not emphasized because "it was not a big problem some years ago", Dr. E. explained. But he also remembered that "many years ago, when I was still a medical student we did not study HIV either, because it was not a problem then. You get my point? Or if you studied it, someone would just hint at it, because the numbers then were so small. But now it is a module at University, it is a full two-months module, where you only learn about HIV. For NCDs we are not there yet. It is better than before but has not yet reached the level of HIV. The medical students only get two lectures on diabetes, 60 minutes each in total, if at all."

Yet another aspect came to the fore in many of the conversations I had with medical personnel and non-medical personnel, diabetes patients and non-diabetes patients alike: the numbers of diabetes must be increasing, because now no matter whom you would ask, everybody knew at least one family member, a friend or a neighbor with diabetes. While before I was told that there were many families without a single person having diabetes, it was now nearly impossible to find anybody who did not have at least one person, an uncle, the grandmother etc. having diabetes: "Before there were many families and you would not find anybody who is diabetic. Now it is very hard to find a family without diabetes. Somehow now so many people have it. That is another angle by the way, that we realize within the members of our family that someone has the disease, which was not there before", a friend once said. It was not only that family members were suffering from diabetes, but it was also the age, which now seemed to decrease: "Those people who are diabetic are above 50 years, I thought. But nowadays there are so many people. I see young people, young girls, young boys, some of them not even ten years old."[22] The experience of a disease, whether one is affected her- or himself or not, takes on a different dimension if it is someone you love who has diabetes. What has before been a narrative, a story one has heard floating somewhere in the distance, becomes visible and personal reality.

The media, too, has its share in contributing to the 'spread' of diabetes in Uganda, Radio shows addressing 'sukali' [diabetes]. I think it must have been at least four times in the three months during my last stay in Uganda, that I heard news about diabetes in the radio (Radio One FM 90). Talks on diabetes, its symptoms and how it could be prevented. Reports on the television, and especially the newspapers that have been increasingly making diabetes a subject in their papers. Searching for the term "diabetes" in the search engine of one of the major Newspapers in Uganda, the New Vision, revealed that while in the year 2000, there was one article published on diabetes entitled "Diabetics hit by insulin shortage", the number of articles published in relation to diabetes had increased up to more than 100 articles in 2016. In the article from 2000 one can read that an estimated 100.000 diagnosed patients would live in Uganda and that Mulago Hospital as well as the Ministry of Health were overwhelmed with "the increasing number of diabetic patients over the last five years." One year later in the same newspaper, on November 15th 2001, there was an article entitled "Diabetes on the Rise" stating that according to health experts "the number of diabetes patients has increased 100 times from 5.000 in 1998 to over 500.000" adding that "the numbers were likely to shoot up due to changes in life style." Yet another eight years later, on the 22nd of November 2009, not only 208 articles had by then been published on diabetes, but an article "Diabetes Mellitus on the increase" reported that two hundred new cases[23] of diabetes would be registered every month in Uganda and the number of cases has reached the two million mark. "Increase" and "rise" are words, which – as we have seen – are verbs often related to diabetes and NCDs and almost used in every article published on diabetes in Uganda and elsewhere. What is repeatedly read in the newspaper finds its way into conversations, and narratives emerge of diabetes as an increasing disease fueled by the observations and experiences an individual makes in the everyday life.

This chapter aimed at positioning NCDs in general and diabetes in specific between the poles of global action, local stagnant policies and guidelines, and the fight

---

22 As hinted at in the previous chapter, type 1 diabetes usually affects young children or adolescents. The perception that diabetes usually affects older people is because there are hardly any distinctions made between these two types and because it is likely that children with type 1 diabetes have often died without having been diagnosed.

23 It does not become clear from the articles where they got these numbers from. The numbers stated in the articles are conflicting. Nevertheless, the message gets clear no matter which numbers are presented: diabetes is on the rise.

for recognition – entangled in a vortex of suspense. Global health claims of dramatically increasing numbers of chronic diseases in countries of the majority world have so far largely contradicted the actions taken to deal with these diseases and the gaps are yet to be filled with comprehensive numerical evidence and funding. We have looked at how NCDs are situated in the global health arena and how they are dealt with on a local level in Uganda. The (global) NCD agenda is getting into its stride, the incorporation of NCDs in the new sustainable development agenda can be seen as one major step of climbing higher up on the global agenda. There is movement and the news of increasing numbers especially of diabetes is spreading. The evidence is there, it is not only numerical, but also, and perhaps even more so, anecdotal. But what counts as evidence today is only that which has been "pushed through the engines of scientific scrutiny [...] and it must speak the language of statistics and epidemiology" (Adams 2013: 56f.). While numerical evidence is still on the top of the hierarchy, other kinds of evidence, anecdotal and observational evidence, may serve as a means to plug the hole where numerical evidence is lacking. It is a way of making sense of increasing numbers, that are hardly visible on paper, a way that becomes real through the lived experiences of individuals in their everyday lives.

"Metrics can be and often are useful", Adams (2013: 225) writes, and in the following chapter we will see that indeed they are, especially in the new global health and what has come to be known as evidence-based medicine (EBM). Yet what has been established as a tool of global health to lead to better and improved health outcomes on a global scale through the application of health interventions, may at the same time lead to exactly the opposite. As Adams states, we "need to recognize what other kinds of work metrics do far beyond their rhetorical claims to improving health" (ibid.). We are best advised to think critically about the use and application of numerical evidence in ways that may not always be the best ways for the people we want to serve and whose lives we want to enhance, as numbers might "generate forms of knowledge and certainty about some things even while effacing others" (ibid.). Next to the push for numbers, a consequence of global health is the impetus to herald in and implement novel technologies (be it ideas, or human and non-human actors). When mentioning global health hereafter, it will not be understood as a straightforward, unproblematic and self-evident notion and field. Instead global health should be treated as a highly complex and heterogeneous phenomenon, which should be handled with careful and critical attentiveness in relation to its moral and ideological reinforcements, paired with the (social, political and technical) consequences it has for health and care. The next chapter intends to lay the conceptual fundament on which I propose the empirical body of this book can be read.

3. Thinking beyond the evident

> Qualitative researchers will continue to narrate local and idiosyncratic lessons from the field, but we must also claim relevance in the highly structured world of intervention trials and evidence-based care. It is the job of social critics to be mindful of the myriad and sometimes unquantifiable forces acting in "evidence" production, especially in places that are under the rationed funding and bureaucratic supervision of governments
> —Smith-Morris 2016: 200.

Technologies without borders?

Technologies in shape of objects, ideas or concepts have always traveled the globe, from one place to the other or spreading from one place to many different places. Technologies today often travel without borders. While they have always traveled to a certain extent, because "that is what they are designed to do" (Hardon 2014: 107), what has over time changed is the scope and rapidity by which technologies are able to travel from and between different contexts and *infrastructures*. A further change is surely the speed by which new technologies emerge, unhesitatingly waiting to voyage in order to improve the lives of or bring satisfaction to their users in one way or the other, ready to replace old and outdated technologies with new models and ideas or innovations. That technologies travel and are sent to travel in the first place is related to their nature as 'travelable' entities, which are as such not necessarily fixed to a specific space and can therefore change places with supposed ease. But their travel is also, and perhaps foremost, related to the assumption that their initial functions and intentions are of use and are used in one way or the other and that they have something to offer to us as human beings (Berg and Timmerman 2003; Nielsen 2010).

The travel of medical technologies intended to be used for a particular purpose – to measure blood glucose levels and enhance health care – is central to understanding the dynamics of why a technology like the glucometer is working and put to work in a certain way in one setting, while it might be working and put to work differently in another. It is the context and the infrastructure(s) of this context that matters and the practices involved in this context against the backdrop of the postcolonial world in which we are living. In this respect, and to make the grade to appreciate and critically involve in any study conducted, the uniqueness of the diverse contexts, the paper by Anderson (2002) entitled 'postcolonial technoscience', invites us to read the 'postcolonial' in technoscience as a "signpost pointing to contemporary phenomena in need of new modes of analysis and requiring new critiques" (Anderson 2002: 643; see also Chakrabarty 2000, Subramaniam et al. 2017). He describes how we have been concerned with studying communities as closed entities for too long instead of viewing the world as a co-production and interrelation of and between different human and non-human actors. It is with a postcolonial perspective with which we may come to see and study this interconnectedness of "changing political economies of capitalism and science, the mutual reorganization of the global and the local, the increasing transnational traffic of people, practices, technologies, and contemporary contests over 'intellectual property'" (Anderson 2002: 643). Pollock and Subramaniam (2016) in turn remind us that it is all too easily forgotten that the history of globalization and all its (inter)related arenas cannot be fully comprehended if we bracket or even obliviate the impacts and dynamics of colonialism and its aftermath.

In accordance to the critiques of other authors (cf. Harding 2009; McEwan 2001) who have challenged a one-way model of technological "diffusion" before, I defy an approach in which science, rationality, progress as well as the creation and innovation of technologies is claimed to derive from the minority world to be disseminated to the majority, so-called non-Western, world (Pollock and Subramaniam 2016; Chambers and Gillespie 2000). In line with the work of Pollock, Subramaniam and colleagues (2016) I intend to follow a "much more mobile, fluid, and dynamic process [...] understood as a set of diversely constituted practices whose movements are too complicated to be captured in simplistic center/periphery frames" (ibid.: 953). The science produced today should be understood as "science in a colonial context" (Seth 2009: 374; Subramaniam et al. 2017). In this sense, this book is situated at the intersections of critical medical anthropology, postcolonial thought and Science and Technology Studies looking at the effects of a global health technology as it travels and arrives in a context with local specificities, as that is what a global technology is eventually about, how it acts and is enacted in practice locally. Or put differently "even while insisting that all practices ultimately act at the local level [they] do global work" (Pollack and Subramaniam 2016: 957).

It is the reality of diabetes (diseases in general) that it is inextricably linked to technology in many ways: the idea and concept of diabetes itself, a chronic disease in nature and therefore opposed to infectious diseases; the global health agenda framing the emergence of non-communicable diseases as a whole and diabetes in specific as a 'global' problem; the (contested) guidelines and standards as to when (which glucose levels) depict diabetes alongside what has come to be known as *evidence-based medicine*, informing 'best' medical practice; the policies put in place by local governments as to how to go about this emerging problem (which are, as we have seen before sometimes missing or stagnant); and above all the medical device, the glucometer, which in fact brings about the evidence of the disease in the first place. All these aspects create part of a global picture of diabetes in the making – notions that travel, the object glucometer that travels and with this an idea of diabetes travels and spreads across the globe to diverse (health) *infrastructures*. As we will see, the travel of technology comes with a transformation of this very technology when it travels as well as when it is applied to a novel context (please note that the travel of a technology does not necessarily have to cross national borders in order to be perceived as traveling) where it will have to be *translated* and engaged with in practice.

Practices hereby, following Mol (2002), is the fundamental analytic entity from which actors, human as well as non-human, emerge. The world does not begin with structure, nor with actors; it does not begin with habitus or with insecurity, but with practice. It begins with incidents that happen and with the movements in everyday life. Entities, humans and things, do not have an inherent and unalterable essence. They can only be the way they are made *in* and *by* a specific local contingent practice. It is only in this sense that they can be examined in a praxiographic way (Mol 2002: 39). Praxiography allows us, but also requires, to take objects and events of any kind into account when trying to study and understand certain phenomena in the world. As an ethnographer, we can never isolate a disease from the practices in which it is enacted, in which technologies make things visible, audible, perceptible and knowable. When isolating objects from the practices in which they are enacted, a body (also glucometer) becomes an independent entity and a reality all by itself (ibid.: 58).

Mol (2002) depicts that knowledge is incorporated in daily events and activities rather than in words, images, books, and privileges practice over principles. An ethnographic study of practices does not search for knowledge inside of subjects but instead locates knowledge primarily in the activities, events, instruments and practices: "Knowledge should not be understood as a mirror image of objects that lie waiting to be referred to. Methods are not a way of opening a window on the world, but a way of interfering with it. They act, they *mediate* between an object and its representations" (Mol 2002: 155; emphasis in the original). In an anthropological understanding of Science and Technology Studies, knowledge and technology are always understood as part of practice, meaning that they can only be understood in their essence through (local) practice for they do not exist outside of it (Mol 2002: 39f). Mol signifies that stability of for instance a clinical diagnosis or a measuring tool is reached through practice, while the production process must be shown through ethnographic research. Knowledge is always also knowledge-practice and situated as such, embedded, located, embodied and inscribed. The same counts for technology: it is shaped by production- and utilization contexts. It is not only about the observation of everyday life and implicit knowledge, but in a fundamental sense it is about practice on an analytical level, and how knowledge and technology can be shaped and determined in a relevant way. In this sense, practice cannot sufficiently be determined with language and discourse, but always has to be observed in the concrete procedure of *being-done*. Hereby it has to be considered that every practice has a historical, social and cultural depth (ibid.: 40) as well as a technological one.

In this following chapter, I attempt to lay the conceptual ground for the empirical chapters – or to say it with the word of Petryna and Biehl (2013), the empirical lanterns of this book – which will follow hereafter. I offer a reading of diabetes and its creation through the conceptual lenses of evidence-based medicine, infrastructures and translation, whereby translation takes place on many different levels: methodologically, historically, conceptually and empirically. By linking these different dimensions to the study of diabetes and its inherent connection to a technological object, the glucometer, I want to picture how diverse actors engage in its use and how each different practice brings about a different kind of knowledge and visibility. I suggest that the study of diabetes and the practices involved to unfold it and make it visible – its diagnosis and testing – is best understood as a complex entanglement of these different spheres by carefully attending to the practices that are at play. While the technologies travel 'borderless', the borders they might face are the borders created for instance by the rigidity of other technologies, such as evidence-based medicine, a high valued tool within the global health of today.

I will link the scholarships of STS and medical anthropology, which may seem problematic upon first sight for they follow different basic assumptions. Anthropologists of technology, have traditionally been interested in studying objects as established, firm and stable in order to understand how this very object is involved in a mutual interference between the object and a culture or societal group. Scholars within STS on the other hand principally intend to understand and 'unblackbox' the scientific and political practices that shape and create objects. Whereas this scholarship repeatedly scrutinizes how the object became what it is and whether exactly this object could become something else – objects are political and could always be something different – they do not perceive objects as firm entities, but as constructed and therefore fluid. Yet what seems problematic and contradictory may at the same time complement each other. By asking the question how the glucometer as a health technology seeks to solve and at the same time create diabetes as a global *and* public health problem in Uganda, both traditions of scholarship may meet fruitfully. By combining the two I intend to make use of the strengths and advantages of these approaches and attempt to plug their respective holes and do what Rockstroh (2007) has done before: merge the high-tech and minority world focus from STS with the capability and expertise of medical anthropology about the majority world and use both to challenge conventional notions and practices within global health.

The rise of evidence-based medicine

In today's world, essential decisions made in the public sphere and the conclusions drawn thereafter, are anticipated to be evidence based. Evidence has a longstanding history in the formation of truth, objectivity and validity. Think of the prominent example of law, where a lack of evidence, a comprehensible proof, may decide whether or not an individual will be convicted. Or what about receiving a receipt when we have made a purchase, which counts as the proof that we have received goods in exchange for money? Evidence proves what is true (or most probable) and what is not; it proves what we have done or not; and it may tell us what to do and what not to do, verified through tangible and convincing scientific methods, and what not. It tells us what *is* and what is *not*. Everything that is not evident allegedly lies outside truth and has no convincing power. As Liebow et al. (2013) state, "[e]ven when it is not obligatory, claiming to be 'evidence based' conveys a sense of legitimacy that many find persuasive" (Liebow et al. 2013: 642).

We have seen that other forms of evidence can be important especially where numerical evidence like in the case of diabetes in Uganda is lacking. It might then be anecdotal evidence (Moore and Stilgoe 2009), which allows us for instance to draw inferences about allegedly rising numbers. Yet it is not this kind of evidence that really counts in what has come to be known as evidence-based medicine (EBM), "the integration of best research evidence with clinical expertise and patient values" (Sacket et al. 2000; see also Brownson et al. 2017). It is numerical, statistical and tangible evidence that has gained momentum in the field of the new global health in this 21st century. There is common consensus that the concept of EBM as we know and understand it today has emerged in the late 1980s/ early 1990s (Timmermans and Kolker 2004; Timmermans and Berg 2003; Timmermans and Mauck 2005; Sackett et al. 1996; n2000)[1] as a response to previously unstandardized and therefore incomparable and hard to assess clinical practices within and across different clinical settings globally. EBM has been established as an approach to endorse a solid "scientific foundation" for a clinical practice that is legitimized by

---

1 Another perception is that EBM has already started developing in the second half of the 19th century with the rise of scientific epistemology achieved through the initiation of the "experimental field" (Adams 2013; Sacket et al. 1996; Gordon 1988; Shapin and Schaffer 2011/1986).

a stronger focus on (new forms of) evidence (Adams 2013). By eliminating the non-uniformity across diverse clinical spaces, a more "conscientious, explicit, and judicious use of current *best evidence* in making decisions about the care of individual patients" (Timmermans and Mauck 2005, as cited in Adams 2013: 55; emphasis in the original) is perceived to not only diminish the asserted problem of unstandardized practices and their outcomes, but to enhance health care delivery and therefore the wellbeing of humans. Standardization hereby is a critical tool of global health. Koch (2016) states that it

> refers to processes by which uniformity is established to promote regulation and an allegedly seamless translation (of goods, statistics, policies, protocols, and so on) across geographical and social boundaries. Anthropologists who study standards and their circulations illuminate how abstract models and technologies travel and become meaningful in specific contexts. These processes are far from value neutral. They are essential for reorganizing medical services in terms of good management, but establishing "good management" in global health is anything but a value-free enterprise, and in this terrain, market values are particularly powerful. (Koch 2016: 52; see also Benatar 2010; Bowker and Star 1999/2015; Lampland and Star 2009; Timmermans and Berg 2003)

EBM is increasingly postulated and endorsed as the golden standard in and for global health interventions, for the assessment of the effectiveness of the treatment of a disease, but also which standards shall be applied and followed in the diagnosis of a disease. What Adams calls the "scientization" of health, that is "Global Health, as new field emerging from the foundation of International Health Development" (Adams 2013: 60) follows the assumption that programs based on EBM will "satisfy the need for more scientific rigor in their international health development efforts. The use of evidence-based medicine will make global health look and feel more scientific because it will *be* more scientific in its practices" (ibid.; emphasis in the original).[2] She contends that the impact of evidence-based medicine has been twofold: first of all, the initiation and creation of an "experimental metrics as a means of providing health care" (see also Petryna 2009) and secondly a shift in how priorities in health care are set in public health in such a way "that 'people [no longer] come first'" (Adams 2013: 54f.; see also Biehl and Petryna 2013; Conalogue et al. 2017). Hereby EBM has transformed into a podium on which truth, accuracy

---

2 According to Goldenberg (2006) evidence-based medicine evolves around five central ideas "first, clinical decisions should be based on the best available scientific evidence; second, the clinical problem, and not the habits or protocols, should determine the type of evidence to be sought; third, identifying the best evidence means using epidemiological and biostatistical ways of thinking; fourth, conclusions derived from identifying and critically appraising evidence are useful only if put into action in managing patients or making health care decisions; finally, performance should be constantly evaluated" (ibid.: 2622; cf. Davidoff et al. 1995).

and reliability can be bought and sold, cleaving off care practices from the people on which they depend and whom they are meant to serve. In different words: EBM is said to have dehumanizing effects, by elevating numbers and statistics above humans and their individual stories, and by pushing guidelines and rules deduced from EBM in front of patient care based on clinical experience and expertise, "turning health workers into rule-followers preoccupied with legalities and the small steps of guidelines instead of active problem solvers aware of holistic patient care" (Adams 2013: 55; Timmermans and Berg 2003).[3]

Randomized controlled trials (RCTs)[4] have increasingly been utilized not only to assess the efficacy of clinical interventions and treatments in terms of their cost-effectiveness, but have at the same time become the basis and at times precondition for the set of priorities, the way disease, its diagnosis and treatment is approached, for policy-making and expenditures in global health, across country-specific health care goals and the way organizations involved work and what they work on (Dehue 2010; Will and Moreira 2010). Questions are sought to be answered such as which medication is to be given to a diabetes patient at what time, in which quantitates for how long it should be taken and following which guidelines? When is it useful or perhaps even harmful to prescribe insulin for an individual with type 2 diabetes? How effective are dietary changes and nutrition strategies for the prevention of diabetes? These are exemplary questions that are and have been addressed through RCTs and have proven to be effective in informing clinical practitioners in their decisions of how to take care of an ailing individual – at least this accounts for care givers in the minority world.

While it is not my aim to condemn evidence-based medicine, I intend to sensitize for and emphasize the fact that any other form of evidence and (medical) practice, which lies outside this golden standard, is seen to stay behind the strength

---

3 As a consequence of the upheld practices and desired outcomes of EBM a "hierarchy of evidence" (Barr et al. 2016; see also Turner 2013; Lambert 2009; Petrisor and Bhandari 2007; Murad et al. 2016) has emerged, ranking different study designs "according to their perceived strength in establishing cause and effect" (Barr et al. 2016: 252). Though evidence can be created in and be based on many different ways of creating what has so many times been labeled truth, in times of evidence-based medicine the golden standard is to draw clinical practice (including interventions) from "the statistical, experimental, and epidemiological model of evidence" (Adams 2013: 55). Resulting from this, any medical practice and intervention that is not based on the best evidence has to be seen as unreliable and consequently of no or only little use in informing policies and guidelines for clinical practice through the eyes of EBM.

4 The randomized controlled trial in evidence-based medicine is a study design that seeks to counteract bias, by randomly choosing and allocating individuals to either one or several medical interventions. Often these groups are divided, one group is e.g. given a placebo, while the other receives a certain pharmaceutical so that the different results can be compared afterwards and the effectivity of the treatment can be assessed (cf. Boruch et al. 2017; Torgerson 2008; Kohn 2014).

and power of EBM by global health actors and the statistical and numerical dogma they prioritize. It is in this approach to healthcare that what counts least, if at all, is what is called anecdotal evidence, ethnographic evidence if you want, which may be especially valuable and even indispensable against the backdrop of little existing or fragmented data, or data that cannot be easily transferred and translated to the realities of a specific setting and attending carefully to the given infrastructures. The local realities are especially important "in situations where health problems are severe and the scarcity of resources makes it vital that they are not wasted" (Chinnock et al. 2005: 0367). Critical voices have further raised concerns about the consequences of emphasizing evidence-based medicine as the global golden standard, for there are great downfalls to it as well. The majority of studies on diabetes for instance has been conducted in places of the minority world, mostly Europe and North America, settings with rather well-off health infrastructures and access to the most up to date laboratory and treatment technology. The data generated under the guise and in the name of evidence-based medicine and global health is not data that derives from deprived health care settings, but from settings in the minority world. How could this evidence inform medical practice in underserved countries where health infrastructures are weak and there is limited or even no access to the newest technology?

According to the best evidence available the use of glucometers is seen as unreliable for the diagnosis of diabetes (and please note that it would surely not be used to diagnose diabetes in any hospital or doctor's office in the minority world). Not only Lovrenčić and colleagues (2013) have concluded that though there are advantages of using glucometers in clinical care and though there are "ongoing improvements in [the] analytical performance [of the glucometer], there is limited evidence on the possible use of [it] for diagnostic purposes [and] their use in the diagnosis of diabetes is not recommended" (ibid.: 2013: 2; cf. Sacks et al. 2011; see also chapter four and any user manual that comes with a glucometer). This point-of-care device, the glucometer, is, however, often the only technology available to the wider public and the only means to uncover the disease and make diabetes visible in Uganda and other countries in the majority world as we will come to see throughout this book. What does this then mean according to the world of evidence-based medicine? Is then any practice, which is not evidence based, or the evidence proves differently a wrong or an insufficient practice?[5]

---

5 The cut-off values that have been determined to categorize the glucose levels of individuals in too high, too low or normal levels, too have been determined in the minority world by, as outlined in chapter one the American Diabetes Association and the International Diabetes Federation though there have been voices that there is a need for different cutoff values for diagnosis "for different ethnic groups" (Smith-Morris 2016: 6).

The power of RCTs as valuable tool in global public health draws from a combination of efficacy and statistical truth for which they are assumed to be "objective (they appear as unbiased, numerical facts) and they are considered valid (they use statistical configurations to present their truths)" (Adams 2013: 57). On the other hand, "[t]he case report counts not for academic promotion, while the randomized controlled trial of thousands of anonymous subjectshas become the lingua franca" in global health (Campo 2006: 1677). Thinking this further means that any 'language' spoken other than the new lingua franca of global health and the practices involved creates nothing more than nice stories that *may* be of relevance, but they also may not. Are the narratives we as anthropologists come to hear and the practices we come to see and observe not reliable, are they not as true as the data generated through RCTs? Is what we do and gather not true 'data', can our insights not be used to establish trustworthy evidence that counts when informing policies, interventions, treatment and diagnostic practices? Again, the upheld golden standard of EBM alongside its RCTs mostly conducted in the minority world and their reliance on all types of metrics will have an influence on what, when and how guidelines may me adjusted (or not) to a specific locality; adjusted to what is there and what is needed. Diabetes is a global health problem that plays out and has to be played out differently in settings with local specificities. I intend to not only describe global health practices with a critical stance, but also demonstrate the relevancy of anthropological knowledge.

RCTs and the decidedly controlled settings in which they are conducted may clearly not be representative of the realities of health care and the people's lives whom they seek to serve and improve and may not relate to the practical needs of the actors involved, such as decision makers (Kelly 2010; Timmermans and Angell 2001). Some have come to term EBM rather pejoratively as 'cook book medicine' or as a 'cook book approach'[6], in order to draw the attention to the dangers and limitations of EBM (see for instance Knaapen 2014; Hawkins 2005). As Adams put it "years of achievements of health policy, not to mention feminism, are summarily cast upon the ash heap of irrelevance here" (Adams 2013: 56). Anecdotal evidence is indeed empirical and might be thought-provoking, but it does not count in the RCT. Evidence-based medicine does not want to rely on the voices of individuals as the main "source of truth [and they] have virtually no purchase, nor do those additional truths garnered from families, communities, or relationships that help form that speech. Certain kinds of evidence are essentially irreconcilable with EBM's definition of reliable evidence, except insofar as such words can be made to fit in

---

6 'Cook book medicine' relates to a clinical practice in which medical practitioners approach individual through guidelines and protocol and not through the attendance of the (medical) needs of an individual (Knaapen 2014).

a quantitative way into the RCT design, or otherwise to corroborate RCT findings with a bit of ethnographic 'color'" (ibid.).

But a major aspect to this is, as Steven Feierman has critically added for consideration, that "all the details of evidence-based medicine assume, as a given, the underlying existence of a set of necessary resources – a body of medical technologies – many of which are unavailable in African settings. What happens to the idea of evidence-based practice when medical resources are not available?" (Feierman 2011, 2017: 171). As Feierman has shown for the case of Ghana and Zimbabwe, not only did the clinical practitioners in each setting and across the settings have different priorities about which disease to address and how certain diseases should be defined. But there was a strong dissatisfaction and frustration with the difficult circumstances and present infrastructures under which they had to perform their jobs. They were constrained to follow 'the best practice' for their local situation – a best practice that had been created elsewhere and was not perceived to be the best for Zimbabwe or Ghana. Though in fact they had a deep knowledge and "realistic understanding of local medical problems", they were lacking the resources to either transform the *global* evidence-based practice into a *local* one or to generate an evidence-based practice, which was able to attend and adapt to the very unique localities (Feierman 2011, 2017: 173). "Local medical knowledge and local leadership deserve special attention at this moment, when so much of the research informing African practice is funded from outside the continent. Most of the research institutions that make key decisions (whether funded by northern-country governments, international organisations or NGOs) are global in scope" (ibid.: 175). Comparable, as we have seen before, with the situation of diabetes in Uganda, where the lack of clinical guidelines and policies hampers and even hinders actions taken to combat diabetes (and other conditions, which are not on the top of the agenda of global health interventions). Respectively, to give a direction of how to proceed, suitable to the resources available. This, as we will see, does not only relate to medical professionals or policy-makers, but also to the individuals who are the ones suffering from a certain disease. The original aim of RCTs, to establish a "fair, robust assessment of the safety, efficacy and effectiveness of a health technology […] is being undermined" (Will and Moreira 2010: 2).

What EBM and its methods seek to diminish, the arbitrariness and unreliability of medical data – which is not based on the results of RCTs – and with this the uncertainty of what can be counted as true evidence, does not reach far down to the individuals who are part of these studies as case numbers. Nonetheless these are the individuals, and populations as a whole, whom country specific health policies, but also global health interventions claim and need to address. Life with a chronic disease like diabetes is uncertain and it remains uncertain even if a correlation between treatment and the effects on the glucose level have been assessed through RCTs. I follow Adams in her assumption that the approaches applied in EBM "have become not just routine but rather tyrannical in the world of clinical health care in the industrialized nations [and elsewhere]" (Adams 2013: 58). Endorsing RCTs and EBM as golden standard has led and is continuing to lead to a prioritization of projects in the public health arena that use these approaches because they are seen to be more reliable and lead to easier evaluations. The rise of EBM has led to a degrading of other forms of evidence. But it is not only an approach adding numbers as ingredients and receiving effectiveness as the outcome, it is an approach fostering the inequality in and across different health care settings and between different diseases instead of diminishing it. As Adams and Biehl aptly write,

> [e]vidence making is, after all, not only the domain of global experts, but an ethical and political proposition that knowledge can come in many forms and be distinctively mobilized. It is a process available to myriad actors as they navigate contemporary medical, humanitarian, and governmental regimes in search of rights and resources. Experiences, often unpredictable, of the social, political, and medical effects of interventions also give rise to new claims of efficacy, new regimes of truth and falsity, and new political and epistemological engagements with outcomes that matter to people. These cumulative experiences form alternative, practice-based forms of evidence that can challenge orthodoxies and perceptual deficits of all kinds and are, in our view, the very fabric of alternative theorizing in global health and beyond. (Adams and Biehl 2016: 124)

It is the spaces in-between, the different practices and how patients and their caregivers will come to enact diabetes and related issues in the practices of every-day life and how they make it visible and knowable in an underserved setting like some of Uganda's governmental health care facilities, which count too. RCTs cannot measure practices, only their outcomes. They cannot capture the practices diverse actors engage in, and the meaning they ascribe to these practices to improve their lives and hold uncertainties at bay. Another aspect goes unquestioned by RCTs: the use of technologies, medical technologies, which are the tools to create (numerical) data and visibility of a disease in the first place. How do their users, medical and non-medical, apply them in their daily practices? What do they come to know with them and produce through them? These are all questions, which I empirically address henceforth. Though statistical data is necessary and even indispensable, anecdotal evidence still matters – or should also matter – in the world of EBM. It is our contribution, even our obligation as anthropologists to give a voice to and picture the individual stories, spaces and practices that fall out of the picture EBM paints. Because these narratives and observations too constitute evidence, even if it is another type of evidence (Adams 2013: 87). As already pointed out in the introduction, with ethnography and the attendance to individuals instead of abstracted numbers I do not aim to block out the 'noise' in order to create uniform descriptions in line with the rigid and statistic nature of RCTs. Instead I intend to highlight them, to break them up, to humanize the statistics and add lived practice and experience to them. The superelevation of EBM in clinical practice has led and will continue to lead to a solidification of a disparity in health priorities where diseases that have been assessed through the methods of EBM will be prioritized over the ones that are not, or not as much. I reason that the less evidence is available in form of statistical data, the more important it becomes to draw on experiences and evidence that is not (only) numerical. The continued focus on EBM and RCTs obscures and hampers the inclusion of practices outside of institutionalized guidelines and protocols.

While I have introduced evidence-based medicine as the main tool for the establishment of evidence in global health today when it comes to the making and in turn acting upon evidence, my work is not about evidence-based medicine per se. Instead, being aware of which claims are made in EBM and how these claims are driven to establish the 'best possible practices' will allow us to have a different view on clinical practices as well as clinical decision making and why they might be performed in a certain way. Practices are at times counteracting (or have to counteract) the best possible evidence. Sometimes practices are exactly not based on the best evidence because there is no available evidence, or this evidence may be fragmented or simply not implemented. It is less about the use of evidence, respectively letting ones' practices be guided by best evidence. Rather, it is about showing that actions are and will be taken even though there is a lack of evidence, or there is no strong evidence, or there might even be counter evidence. Ultimately what may be perceived as best practice in one setting, is not necessarily the best practice in another setting, especially because there are different evidences and because (health) infrastructure matters.

Infrastructures or "Stuff, staff, space and systems"

"I have just returned from Liberia with a group of physicians and health activists. We are heading back in a few days. The country is in the midst of the largest ever epidemic of Ebola haemorrhagic fever [...]. The Ebola virus is terrifying because it infects most of those who care for the afflicted and kills most of those who fall ill [...]. [It] was known that the virus could be transmitted as the result of a failure to follow the rules of modern infection control: the nurses reused needles and did not wear gloves, gowns or masks, which were all in short supply. Nor did the nurses, still less their patients, receive what in Brussels, Boston or Paris would count as modern medical care [...]. Any emergency room in the US or Europe can offer such care, and can also treat patients in isolation wards [...]. Properly equipped hospitals are even scarcer than staff, and this is true across the regions most affected by Ebola. Also scarce is personal protective equipment

(PPE): gowns, gloves, masks, face shields etc. In Liberia there isn't the staff, the stuff or the space to stop infections transmitted through bodily fluids, including blood, urine, breast milk, sweat, semen, vomit and diarrhoea [...]. But the fact is that weak health systems, not unprecedented virulence or a previously unknown mode of transmission, are to blame for Ebola's rapid spread. Weak health systems are also to blame for the high case-fatality rates in the current pandemic [...]. The obverse of this fact – and it is a fact – is the welcome news that the spread of the disease can be stopped by linking better infection control (to protect the uninfected) to improved clinical care (to save the afflicted). An Ebola diagnosis need not be a death sentence. Here's my assertion as an infectious disease specialist: if patients are promptly diagnosed and receive aggressive supportive care – including fluid resuscitation, electrolyte replacement and blood products – the great majority, as many as 90 per cent, should survive [...]. Without staff, stuff, space and systems, nothing can be done." (Farmer 2014)

The words stated above are not my words, but the words of the anthropologist and physician Paul Farmer, a reflection of his trip to Liberia in the middle of the Ebola crisis in 2014 – as Farmer states "the largest ever epidemic of Ebola haemorrhagic fever". The Ebola crisis in West-Africa, affecting several countries, lasted for nearly two years, and claimed the lives of thousands of people. It might come as a surprise to you why I open with this reflection, when this book is ultimately about diabetes. Unlike Ebola, diabetes is neither infectious nor is it a threat to the health of the global public in the sense that a virus 'migrates' from one person to another or from primates to humans or vice versa. No country will have to shut down its borders due to increasing numbers of diabetes like it was the case for Ebola. Indeed, these diseases are fundamentally different in terms of their nature, transmission and the care they require (long-term care vs. emergency care). Chronic diseases are dichotomized with infectious diseases. Whereas diseases generally come along with medical dependency, regression and, if a suitable treatment is implemented, with recovery, chronic diseases have a restricted prospect of recovery, a longer period of medical dependency and regression. The course of chronic diseases is uncertain and its duration unlimited. The treatment can alleviate the pains and symptoms, but there is no cure (Scandlyn 2000: 131; see also chapter one).

Yet there are similarities between the two diseases, when they occur in countries of the majority world: a failure to offer what Farmer (2014) calls "modern medical care", guiding all practices by the 'best' available evidence; health systems that are perceived to be weak; and the fact that both diseases could allegedly be handled differently if they were to befall Europe or other parts of the minority world, where there is more of "staff, stuff, space and systems". Accordingly, care is inseparably linked to technology. Care in turn is practice: it involves "doctoring" and nursing, handling of technology and applying it correctly (Mol 2008). As I would like to add, caring also involves making disease visible for it is not only inextricably linked to technology (such as EBM as the standard and guideline, as well as a [traveling] medical device to uncover disease), but also to the infrastructures in which these practices take place.

If the Ebola crisis has lead health researchers and practitioners to come to one main conclusion, then it might be that the crisis has unraveled and made visible one thing, which seemingly lurks unrecognized as long as it 'works': health infrastructure. As Alice Street points out in her talk "Rethinking Infrastructures for Global Health" at the University of Edinburgh in 2014[7], infrastructure is something that is not present consciously, but happens in the background of our daily lives. Infrastructure is what enables us to drive a car, to draw money from our bank accounts, to take a shower. It is what "causes our economies to work and our societies to function" (Street 2014a) and there is hardly any reason why we should question infrastructure as long as it is functioning, working, and keeps the society in which we are living going. When infrastructure, however, is not working or not as we are used to, when the roads on which we want to drive our cars decay, the automated teller from which we want to draw money has broken down or the water pipes stay dry, what we have been taking for granted before becomes visible and in turn questioned due to its 'failure'.[8] When actors attempt to practice evidence-based medicine in a space of uncertainty, then a space of institutional poverty followed by overcrowded hospitals, lacking resources and lacking access will require different actions. As Alice Street writes "[u]ncertainty provokes improvisation and sustains hope in future well-being, personal transformation, and national development. But the hospital is also a place where failure is frequently experienced as the endpoint of hope, where people [...] discover they are socially invisible – unrecognized as a person in their relationships with doctors, kin, the state, or the networks of global science" (Street 2014c: 19). It is then when we come to question infrastructure.

But, to take the wind out of the sails, I will not offer you a clear definition of what infrastructure really *is*. Rather I want to direct our attention towards (health) infrastructure and think about what it might mean in an already 'unstable' place, when "[b]iomedical ways of knowing, and the objects biomedical practitioners seek to render visible, remain inherently unstable" (Street 2014c: 225). What happens when a global health technology travels and arrives in a new, local, setting? What do we understand as stable or unstable coming from a background with rather well-

---

7 The talk can be accessed online: https://www.youtube.com/watch?v=HehA7XmUzHM.
8 Instead of emphasizing the 'invisible nature' of infrastructures, though in fact the materiality of infrastructure forbids to name it this way, Brian Larkin (2013) notes that infrastructures are not as unnoticed and taken for granted, "but instead they inhabit a whole spectrum of visibilities, from opacity to spectacle" (Harvey et al. 2017: 3).

functioning health care infrastructures? To repeat the words of Paul Farmer (2014) "[w]ithout staff, stuff, space and systems, nothing can be done" (see also Beisel 2014). Street (2014b) elaborates on his thought that "where there is no running water, no ambulances, no gloves or protective clothing, and few health workers or laboratories, what seems easy elsewhere becomes exceedingly difficult, and thousands of lives are lost" (ibid.). Health infrastructures not only become visible, when something is missing, but it is infrastructure, which influences the ways in which what is already there – knowledge, technologies, space and stuff – as well as that what arrives anew, like traveling technologies – is and can be handled and how knowledge is generated accordingly. It is infrastructure in which technologies are embedded and enacted, and it is also in this frame, where (medical) practices take place.

As hinted at, to define infrastructure is an exceedingly difficult undertaking for it is the perspective from which infrastructure is studied and viewed that influences the ways in which we may come to a definition. This difficulty, however, is at the same time the strength of the notion of infrastructure, for it is flexible, dynamic and not static. As Harvey et al. (2017) infer, "[o]nce we approach infrastructures as dynamic and emergent forms, it is clear that we cannot specify their contours in advance. The question 'what is infrastructure' must therefore be addressed, and experimented with, in registers at once conceptual and empirical" (ibid.: 5). Infrastructure can be everything and related to every-thing and everyone: to roads (Beck et al. 2017); to the connections and networks between people (Simone 2004) or to classification systems (Bowker and Star 1999); the built networks, which enable goods, people and ideas to travel (Larkin 2013); or to health infrastructures (Street 2014) and the practices involved. They seem to reside somewhere and every-where between practice and structure. Harvey et al. (2017) suggest a definition of infrastructure stating that we

> are dealing with technologically mediated, dynamic forms that continuously produce and transform socio-technical relations. That is, infrastructures are extended material assemblages that generate effects and structure social relations, either through engineered (i.e. planned and purposefully crafted) or non-engineered (i.e. unplanned and emergent) activities. Seen thus, infrastructures are doubly relational due to their simultaneous internal multiplicity and their connective capacities outwards. (ibid.: 5)

In this sense infrastructure itself becomes a technology, yet not bound to sheer materiality but emerging from and through practices and their interpretations and are thus relational (Calkins and Rottenburg 2017: 254; cf. Pinch 2010). Accordingly, infrastructure might be best understood and studied in context as a concept, which always stands in relation to something and/or somebody.

In her rich ethnography of a public hospital in Papua New Guinea, Alice Street (2014c), too, refers to infrastructure as a relational technology, which, though fragile, provides novel and unforeseen ways to make humans visible and knowable (ibid.). Harvey et al. (2017) point at an important aspect of infrastructure: we will never know which kind of infrastructure will matter and be perceived as relevant in people's lives and it will not "allow us to know just where or how radically new forms of infrastructure might emerge as significant forces" (ibid.: 6).

In line with Harvey et al. (2017), I propose to read infrastructure alongside its diverse possibilities "looking for those underlying configurations that are not necessarily the site of active reflection on the part of those whose lives they shape, while also attending to the ways in which people do sometimes reflect on the socio-material conditions that shape their life worlds" (ibid.: 5). Infrastructure is a process as well as it is an achievement, it can be a motor as well as an impediment to transformation (Star and Ruhleber 1996), it can be visible to some while remaining invisible to others. Whereas earlier studies on infrastructure (Bowker 1995; Star and Ruhleder 1996; Star 1999) focused on the steadiness and firmness of infrastructure (Calkins and Rottenburg 2017), I want to highlight the dual character of infrastructures as material manifestations as well as their fluidity in terms of the connections and flows they enable between people and technologies. As Calkins and Rottenburg (2017) put it "infrastructures are not clearly bounded entities out there but relational configurations that unfold from practices and interpretations (e.g. Pinch 2010). They are networks that are inscribed with theories about their usage and users and yet are often put to other uses than their designers anticipated (Akrich 1992)" (Calkins and Rottenburg 2017: 254).

Why infrastructures 'fail', can have various reasons. There can be disturbances coming from the inside, like an Ebola virus, or external disruptions such as traveling technologies entering unknown terrain. Unlike, for instance, traveling technologies like the Rapid Diagnostic Test (RDT), which has specifically been designed for places with 'weak' infrastructures and for places with limited access to e.g. power and other resources etc.[9], the glucometer is a truly global technology in the sense that it can be found anywhere across the globe, as diabetes occurs everywhere. Yet its use may vary according to the infrastructural givenness. A weak health infrastructure is understood to hamper evidence-based medicine and the practices involved (Lhachimi et al. 2016; Al-Gelban et al. 2009; Agarwal et al. 2008). Calkins and Rottenburg (2017) have introduced the term "infrastructure of evidence", the production of evidence as "a specific form of infrastructuring that connects politics, science, technologies, and objects [...] and human bodies" (Calkins

---

9 This is not to say that the RDT functions and can be put to work without problems occurring. It is rather to make the point that an RDT has been designed for a very specific context – with weak infrastructures, as opposed to the glucometer.

and Rottenburg 2017: 254). Practices within this frame are guided by the prevailing infrastructures as well as they shape them. In this sense, a traveling technology is embedded in infrastructures which enable practices, as well as they may hamper them. It is a constant interplay between infrastructures as stable networks and infrastructures as fragile systems. The production of evidence through and around it can lead to new forms of infrastructure (ibid.: 262). I argue that a traveling technology like the glucometer may bring stability in one setting and fragility to another, or evoke both at the same time even in the same place.

While evidence and the production thereof may be certain, it can sometimes be disputable, or, as mentioned before, it can be lacking. This is one part of the explanation for why some traveling technologies – like evidence-based medicine –play out differently in different contexts (Freeman 2009; Czarniawska and Sevón, 2005), respectively has to be played out differently according to the infrastructural context. It then becomes a matter of translation, for "if technologies do not work autonomously, then it is the relationships between stuff, space, people and systems that matter" (Street 2014). Translations that take place in a certain setting, with a specific infrastructure, which enables and informs practices. Translation has especially been utilized among researchers and practitioners in relation to knowledge transfer or the translation of evidence into practice in the field of healthcare (Freeman 2009). It is in this area where the findings of health research have addressed infrastructural failure to adequately and sustainably translate research findings into clinical practice and policy making.

Translation(s) in a technologized world

There is one core reason why we as anthropologists should think about technologies in our theoretical and empirical endeavors: we live in a technologized world in which the way we perceive our lives is influenced, framed and reframed, defined and redefined by our interactions with the technologies in our everyday lives in the one way or the other. Accordingly, the ways in which we relate to matters of health and disease and how we experience them may change when (new) (biomedical) technologies are applied. This is also one of our hopes – that we can improve a condition or maintain it with the technologies that are available, the ones we have access to, and are therefore able to make use of it (Casper and Koenig 1996). While we include this 'technological gaze' (Crawford 2017) in our empirical and ethnographic studies, Hardon and Moyer (2014) point out, we need to integrate "the creative agency of the users of medical technologies, the particularities of local markets and care constellations, class hierarchies, social relations and family dynamics. As biomedical technologies are resisted, reinvented and adopted, they shape and reinforce site-specific constellations of care, social and family relationships, and class and inter-generational structures of power" (ibid.: 112; see also Hardon 2016).

Technological devices share the commonality that they have a specific purpose and an intended use, we utilize them in order to reach something and to arrive at a certain point that might be better than the point from which we have departed (Akrich 1992; Mol 2002). They have been designed and created to serve a very specific goal and often for a very specific group of people. Technological devices are never isolated but instead emerge through a web of networks, which include human as well as non-human actors. All together are needed to get them started, keep them going, and to make them stable (Akrich 1992: 205). In order to become stable, technological devices have to be embedded in a set of infrastructural predispositions in order for them to fulfill their duty. Or, as I suggest, technologies can be seen as being embedded in infrastructure(s), which determine the way in which this technology can be handled, utilized and translated. It is in the realm of infrastructure in which an envisioned duty or purpose of a technology may become visible as (what has often been termed) failed or altered.

Following Akrich (1992) every technology is based on a script, which has arisen in and through the development of its design and creation. When a technology is envisaged and consequently designed and 'manufactured' a "large part of the work of innovators is that of *inscribing* this vision of (or predictions about) the world in the technical content of the new object", with a final product, which she refers to as "script" (Akrich 1992: 208; emphasis in the original). When a designer or innovator creates a technology, she has a pre-defined set of actors in mind – their competencies, motives, aspirations etc. These actors will put this technology to use in a defined space, as for instance a hospital. The designer will carefully think about the shape, color and the functions of the technology in order to hit the right savor of its prospective users, which will make them aspire to have it (ibid.). Technologies thus follow certain scripts, whereby the technology itself also constitutes the interaction between technology and user in a certain manner: "Like a film script, technical objects define a framework of action together with the actors and the space in which they are supposed to act" (ibid.: 209).

When reading about technology or knowledge transfer, especially when it concerns the travel of a technology from the minority world to the majority world, there is often the talk of how difficult it is to move them from one place to the other. De Laet writes that "the very phrase 'technology and knowledge transfer', after all, suggest[s] that we are talking about thoughts and things that move from place *a* to place *b* that is, in significant respects, different from place *a*. The phrase suggests that these technologies and knowledges cross a line" (de Laet 2002: 1; emphasis in the original). Madeleine Akrich (1993) has for example displayed how a technology, which was meant to generate power, the 'gazogene', has failed to continue doing its work because it was fired using a kind of wood to which it was not geared. Critical voices have noted that the inscription process at time tends to have a marginalizing and excluding effect. With their work, Fishman et al. (2017) want to depict and draw critical attention to the complex entanglement surrounding issues of race, nation ethnicity, class and related spheres of inequality that come along with and become visible through the production and practices of technoscientific knowledge. Working on gendered and sexual dimensions of technologies and their design they state that in the process of inscription technologies may become "identity projects and through [the] study of their inscription reveal how hegemonic ideals [...] of difference emerge and become stable" (ibid.: 389; see also Felt 2017). Inscription is accordingly never only a well-intended procedure in the development of a technology, but may entail exclusion. While the designer and creators of technology have certain visions in mind, there will always be humans who will use the technology, which they haven't been thinking about before. Likewise, there will be humans who will put a technology to use in a place that was not insinuated before and used for a purpose that was not anticipated before.

But no matter how a technology will be put to use – sometimes according to, sometimes against projected scripts – the concept of technology suggests that devices of all sorts have to be enabled in the first place. Enabling is, however, not restricted to technological artefacts, but involves the organizational and institutional structures –infrastructures – to which these devices may be connected and in which they are meant to be embedded, as well as the epistemic and normative suppositions they implicate. Nonetheless, technology is reliant on those human beings who (want to) put them to use, who do or are expected to do something with them, who live and interact with them in their daily lives. Technology is never a passive tool but a constituent part of networks tying human and non-human actors together. To enable a technology and unfold the script, as soon as it leaves its place of origin and creation, and in order to get adapted and appropriated, a traveling (medical) device must be translated and this in often unforeseen ways (Hardon and Moyer 2014).

In line with Michel Callon's 'sociology of translation' (Callon 1986), translation can be understood as a process of shifting an ontologically different element into a stable network, a web of arrangements. When technologies, or medical devices for that matter, travel, new institutional engagements might have to be put in place to cope with the impacts of the device and to keep it going, to keep it stable or to make it stable again – to follow the intention it was made for or create it anew. As Callon points out, human and non-human actors are not only individual entities, but instead they comprise a whole set of different networks involving institutional realities as well as (infrastructural) materialities. They maneuver between technological, social as well as cultural realities and ontologies (ibid.). With his renown example of the revival of the scallops in Brittany, France, applying a cultivation system commonly used in Japan, Callon shows that every translation involves a process[10]. He describes: "The scallops are transformed into larvae, the larvae into numbers, the numbers into tables and curves which represent easily transportable, reproducible, and diffusable sheets of paper [...]. The scallops have been displaced. They have been transported into the conference room through a series of transformations" (Callon 1986: 217f.). Callon specifies that actors are not apprehended as individual humans, but are coalesced to a network of discourses, institutional and material infrastructures, technologies, policies and their implementation, standardizations and so on. All aspects together influence the way in which we as human beings perceive the world, and it controls but also secures the way we behave and think (ibid.).

The concept of translation has found entrance into diverse fields of academia as well as organizations and is utilized especially among those who are studying or working with the transfer of knowledge, like in the field of health care and health systems research.[11] Freeman (2009) denotes that "[w]hat is translated often seems somehow inferior, not real or original" (ibid.: 430). Translation, however, can be the spectacles with which we can take

> closer attention to the problem of shared meaning and how it might be developed. It seems to represent some new epistemological lubricant, facilitating the dissemination of texts and the application and use of the knowledge and information they contain. Simply, translation might be the key to transfer. Yet when we stop to think, we are more ambivalent. What is translated often seems somehow inferior, not real or original. (ibid.: 430)

According to Latour translations are always strategic undertakings and argues that in the process of translating a technology into a more customary shape, some things get 'lost in translation' (Latour 1987; 1999). I follow the assumption that traveling, or moving a technology from one place to another, will not only transform the technology and require (re)interpretation but it will influence the receiving context[12] alongside its infrastructures as well as its actors (Macamo and Neubert 2008;

---

10 Callon calls the different phases of the process of translation: problematization, interessement, enrolment and mobilization. He investigates how a network of relationships (actor-network) is formed through 'equivalences', which lead to translation(s) (Callon 1986; Freeman 2009).
11 The World Health Organization for instance has come to speak of knowledge translation (KT) as "a paradigm to address many of the challenges and start closing the "know-do" gap. [it is defined as] [t]he synthesis, exchange, and application of knowledge by relevant stakeholders to accelerate the benefits of global and local innovation in strengthening health systems and improving people's health (http://www.who.int/ageing/projects/knowledge_translation/en/).
12 In the case of diabetes, technology does not only contribute to the uncovering and monitoring of the disease, but also contributes to the generating of numbers and therefore the "making of diabetes" epidemiologically.

de Laet and Mol 2000). I want to argue that while something gets lost, something else might be won at the same time. Instead of relating to translation and everything that is deviant of its alleged intended use as failure, I instead want to steer the view towards translation that leads to gains on many different sides. It is less about judging that the glucometer is used differently than rather pointing to the fact that with certain translations certain things can be gained that might in the end be more beneficial. Translation is always an active act, which involves getting the best out of a technology for a specific purpose, in a specific setting and at a specific time.

As hinted at before when a technology embarks on a journey or is sent to travel it is implicitly, sometimes explicitly, nurtured by the assumption that it will be adapted to a new context, that the actors will embrace it and tap into its use, without problems occurring. Anthropological approaches to this very moment of adaptation, to the "local" ways of using a technology alien to the receiving context, can especially be found in studies and debates on appropriation. Appropriation is the process of actively "making something to become one's own" (Hahn 2008: 195), forming, taming and subjugating it according to ones needs and expectations (Hahn 2008; Müller-Rockstroh 2007; Spittler 2002; Beck 2001). Making a technology one's own may involve changing the intended locality of its use, the time of its use, but also the actors who use it or the purpose for what it is used.

A much-cited article on the changing capability and adaptability of a technology is the striking work of de Laet and Mol (2000), who vividly describe the travel and appropriation of the Bush Pump 'B' type to Zimbabwe and how it is, can be and must be reconfigured in order to 'work', though there is not only one way of working, but rather "grades and shades of 'working'; there are adaptations and variants" (ibid.: 226). While the material with which it has been built is firm, its boundaries are what de Laet and Mol refer to as vague and not clear fixed, but as 'fluid' (ibid.). They state that

> [p]erhaps in this it [the Bush Pump] is like the clinical diagnosis of anaemia in medicine which, unlike its laboratory-based cousin, reveals a flexibility that allows it to travel almost anywhere. As has been argued elsewhere, the adaptability of clinical diagnostic methods suggests that they hold together as a fluid, rather than as a network. Something similar might be true for other technologies that transport well. Therefore we mobilize the metaphor of the fluid here to talk of the Bush Pump. In doing so we hope to contribute to an understanding of technology that may be of help in other contexts where artefacts and procedures are being developed for intractable settings which urgently need working tools. Because in traveling to 'unpredictable' places, an object that isn't too rigorously bounded, that doesn't impose itself but tries to serve, that is adaptable, flexible

and responsive – in short, a fluid object – may well prove to be stronger than one which is firm. (de Laet and Mol 2000: 226)

As Müller-Rockstroh puts it "appropriation includes acquiring skills and experience as to how, when and where to use a technology and what for" (Müller-Rockstroh 2007: 9), but also who uses it and why and what has to be done in order for it to 'work' in one way or the other. Time, space and purpose, as well as the user(s) are hereby interconnected. The process of appropriation, adaptation and translation involves a dismantling of things in one moment while rebuilding and reconfiguring them in the next and with this creating new ways of using as well as understanding the technology. While technologies travel, it is important to note that though they are not bound to a certain space, they are, however, bound to a certain time and often to a predefined group of humans. Technologies seldom stay the same, they change over time due to (medical and technological) innovation and progress. What is then presented is always a picture given for a very specific point in time. In the case of the glucometer you will come to see that the models and types of glucometer available on the market for instance are changing rapidly even within a short period of time. As Müller-Rockstroh states

> [a]cknowledging the transformative capacity of technology, however, brings with it the question of how technology then can be assessed. If technology and objects change as they travel, yet are at the same [time] made to travel in order to do certain kind[s] of things, for instance to solve urgent health problems, technology assessment has to capture this technology 'in the making'. (Müller-Rockstroh 2007: 3)

Yet there is another dimension to this work: the very technology that is made to solve public health issues, the glucometer, which is intended to measure glucose values of an individual and support self-monitoring activities, is – in Uganda and elsewhere – at the same time the technology that creates and helps to shape this global public health problem. In other words: without the glucometer, it becomes difficult and, in some places, even impossible to solve anything at all. There is a double function of the glucometer in a setting like Uganda: while it is meant to solve a problem, it is at the same time the means that supports in creating this (public health) problem – the creation of diabetes as a health issue, which, as opposed to the longstanding perceptions, is not only a problem in other places of the minority world, but exactly also in Uganda. This field of tension offers us a beautiful example of a technology that becomes a different technology in a different place and even within the same country, because it travels and because it is changed through the practices, which it brings to the fore and in which it is involved. "The transfer of expertise […] is predicated on a labor of translation. How a technology moves from context to context, and what travels with it and what stays behind is thus an open question" (von Schnitzler 2013: 679; cf. Rottenburg 2009) and therefore becomes an empirical matter.

In what follows I explore the effects of a traveling health technology in its implementation and application to a receiving context empirically. We will meet the glucometer as a contraption, that indeed is flexible, fluid and 'travelable' in nature, yet it also has boundaries. The glucometer is neither strikingly beautiful nor can spare parts be replaced when they break. In fact, the whole glucometer, transforms into a useless object (you might call it waste), when something breaks. The following empirical chapters introduce the glucometer as a paradox object. Evidence-based medicine is a rigid and narrow concept, which allegedly does not allow much room for creativity and deviation in order to count as good practice. The glucometer hereby acts twofold: it is a means to follow, but also to distort the rigidity of this concept and the practices involved. It is a tool to deliver evidence in Uganda, while it at the same time is perceived to be an unreliable object. This paradox object will be the protagonist of each of the four following chapters, involved in different practices and therefore bringing about a different glucometer and making a different aspect of diabetes in Uganda visible.

4. A 'simple' technology and its translations: the glucometer[1]

> Technical objects and people are brought
> into being
> in a process of reciprocal definition
> in which objects are defined by subjects
> and subjects by objects
> ——Akrich 1992: 222.

There are different reasons for why we might purchase a glucometer. The most obvious one is that we buy a glucometer when we or a family member has been diagnosed with diabetes. We will be confronted with an abundance of different brands and types of glucometers. Yet, as the logic of choice suggests, there will be a technology that will suit our taste, the needs and wishes we might have for a technology that is meant to make our daily lives easier and more convenient (Mol 2008). Once we have decided, which glucometer we want to have, we will pay a certain amount of money (the price for a glucometer varies substantially, ranging

---

[1] An earlier version of this chapter has been published in a coauthored article with Uli Beisel (Liggins and Beisel 2017). The article published previously has aimed at giving an overview of different claims stated in the glucometer manual and how they are translated when the glucometer is put to use in Uganda (the claim that it is made for the daily self-monitoring of diabetes patients; secondly that it makes the life of its user easier and finally that it should not be used for the diagnosis of diabetes). In order to make the article useful and therefore contribute to the research question on what the glucometer in Uganda can actually make visible, you will find this chapter extended and fundamentally restructured and enriched with further empirical material. Though there are similarities in the overall argument and conceptual approach, namely to think aspects of translation together with matters of care, this chapter especially focuses on the claim that the glucometer is not be used for the diagnosis of diabetes – alongside the impracticabilities and challenges a user in Uganda might face when wanting to use the device for diagnostic purposes. Put into context of the research question of what a traveling technology like the glucometer, as it is applied to a context with weak health infrastructures can actually make visible, the empirical material in this chapter contributes to the enhancement of the argument in novel ways. I have added a detailed description of the glucometer itself as well as I have added experiences and challenges of more actors in the field, such as the perspectives of biomedical engineers, and with this a more profound insight into the glucometer its use, perception and translation.

from 11 USD up to 180 USD, excluding the testing strips[2]). In return, we will receive a small cardboard box, protecting the glucometer and the supplies that come with it, from external damage. Usually a "starter-box" contains the glucometer, some blood lancets (needed to prick the finger), and around ten glucose strips, on which a drop of blood has to be applied so that the machine can start measuring the amount of glucose in our blood. That is the main purpose of the machine: measure the amount of glucose in the blood and produce a number, which we can read and interpret as deviation or as compliance with glucose level standards. This means, this very number tells us whether or not our glucose level is too high, too low or just right.

The previous part of the book has established a conceptual background against which the empirical body can be read. This chapter explores and focuses on the technological device that is used for measuring glucose levels and yields the diagnosis of diabetes: the glucometer. As mentioned before, the glucometer is the first-choice (as often the only choice) technology when it comes to diagnosing and testing diabetes in Uganda in most governmental health facilities. Considering its practicability and appearance, the glucometer has undergone some major transformations. From a former bulky machine that was kept stationary at doctors' offices, to a now small device, which can easily fit in one's pants pocket. Today, glucometers are widely spread and are not only used in doctors' offices, but also in the homes of individuals with diabetes. This holds especially true for the minority world, where a glucometer can be found in nearly every home of individuals with diabetes, and often even more than one. As glucometers are no longer bound to one place, they can accompany individuals wherever they to go or decide to take them. They come in different shapes, sizes, colors, with different prices, and with diverse functions.

As a so-called point-of-care device – a device which delivers quick results, is easy to use and can also be applied outside the hospital setting – the glucometer has been designed and produced for (self-)monitoring practices of individuals with diabetes. That is, by purchasing a glucometer that suits one's needs, an individual who is diagnosed with diabetes may engage in measuring the glucose level outside of the clinical setting (compare chapter six). Although it is meant to facilitate the management and handling of diabetes, the consequences of its use may be surprising and do not always make things easier. In order to understand the impact of this technology, we will take a deeper look at it in this chapter. Being produced, 'inscribed' and described by privatized and well-funded markets of Europe, the US, and Asia, the technology is put to use in a setting alien to its country of origin.

---

2   The small size of most glucometers makes them suitable for an easy travel across countries. Glucometers come into Uganda from all parts of the world, sometimes as gifts from family members when they have traveled abroad, sometimes as donations. We will get back to this point later.

Following the narration of the previous chapter, a technology is made and remade, is built and rebuilt in the process of its appropriation, adaption and translation, and thus creates novel ways of using and understanding it. Hereby not only the user of the technology and contexts of its application changes, but also the traveling device may change. Technologies are never static entities. They are fluid in the process and a result of their translation (Mol and De Laet 2000). In some ways, the glucometer is an "immutable mobile" in the way Latour insinuated. It is a truly global diagnostic device that enables scientific data to travel while the results stay the same. In other words, it enables the standardization of diagnosis.

Whereas this is the case in theory, the realities of the glucometer in use are more complex and not as straightforward. As we will see, the glucometer can be understood as a fluid technology (Mol and De Laet 2000). It transforms fundamentally in purpose, from being a device designed for the self-monitoring of patients into a means of primary diagnosis of diabetes in Uganda. Although the materiality of the device stays the same, the translation brings about a different glucometer (cf. Esguerra and Berger 2017). This difference, or transformation, can be read as a beneficial process. More patients can be diagnosed with diabetes in Uganda's impoverished health system. However, the creative adaptation of the device is risky, perhaps even dangerous. If only tested with the glucometer, the risk of false diagnoses due to the error-proneness of glucometers might increase (Klonoff and Prahalad 2015). That a technology is prone to error, however, is nothing that can be seen with bare eyes but instead requires the use of further, more complex machineries that are able to uncover these errors. In an impoverished health setting it is often an impossible endeavor. Additionally, testing strips are a scarce and expensive commodity. The primary diagnosis of diabetes with a glucometer is therefore all but a given in Uganda's health system. This means that a glucometer is indeed not a straightforward product, as its designers might have imagined, but rather an ambivalent achievement (Beisel and Schneider 2012).

Following Law, "to translate is to make two words equivalent. But since no two words are equivalent, translation also implies betrayal [...]. It is about moving [things] around, about linking and changing them. In short, translation is always insecure, a process susceptible to failure. Disorder – or other orders – are only precariously kept at bay" (Law 2007: 5). Therefore, I suggest, one needs to complement a focus on translation with a focus on care. That being said, the process of translation is incremental in health systems with ailing infrastructures. Even the transfer of the best technology cannot function as a (quick) fix. Caring for diabetes patients in Uganda is also a tinkering and consequently requires the glucometer to be used creatively. It involves to be translated in the various ways, which will be documented below. This also means that the glucometer itself needs to be seen as a fluid technology of care, and not of patient choice (Mol 2008). In Uganda, it is rather a matter of accessing a glucometer in the first place, respectively having to take what is available on the market or given to a health center, than satisfying a certain taste or individual needs. It is not a matter of choice, but of access, as will be described in more detail soon.

Cartwright, referring to Annemarie Mol and her colleagues (2010) who introduced a novel way of augmenting the notion of care with the notion of tinkering, describes

> how people use technologies in unexpected ways while caring for the unexpected. Tinkering occurs as caregivers make adjustments and compromises when the rigid protocols of biomedicine need to be enacted in emergencies or in cases where the necessary accoutrements of medicine are not available. As one moves further and further out from large, well-resourced hospitals and clinics, to settings where even the simplest of technologies are often not available, such tinkering becomes even more important. (Cartwright 2016: 175)

While in a capitalist logic of patient choice, the availability of glucometers would be seen as sufficient, I follow Mol's argument (2008). I suggest, in line with my proposition in the conceptual chapter, that we must carefully analyze the practices of use and dis-use of the glucometer in order to transform it into a technology of care and dissect its fluidity. In order to translate it in ways that help to improve people's lives and translate it into a technology of care that does not just end up in the 'glucometer graveyard' in hospital cabinets and patient homes. It must be translated into a technology that actually functions and is adjusted to the needs of both, the Ugandan public health system and individuals' lives.

This chapter will take the translation(s) of the glucometer, the betrayals or failures as they are often called, as point of departure. Originally thought of as a facilitator of self-monitoring practices in the minority world, the device traveled to the Ugandan health system where it is responsible for diagnosing and testing patients of an entire health center and even beyond. We will see that the glucometer, as it is applied in an unprepared and impoverished health care system, may evoke irritation rather than facilitation. I intend to show how the introduction and translation of global health technologies for a disease like diabetes may only slowly contribute to the development of novel infrastructural and political engagements on the ground. Approaching the issue through the conceptual lens of translation will help us to challenge more conventional notions of a unilateral technology transfer and social engineering. It will further relate these processes to aspects of (un)changing institutions and broader questions of social (dis)order. Instead of viewing the creative translation of the glucometer as failure or maladaptation, I suggest that a flexible translation is part of an essential process that keeps care practices going (see also Liggins and Beisel 2017).

Glucometer user manuals will serve as a starting point. I have chosen to introduce some of their descriptions and connected claims to highlight their (dis)embeddedness in the Ugandan context and to critically examine, whether the promises are kept, broken or transformed. These promises are formulated by designers and producers and are manifested in a small booklet. We will see that using and/or owning a glucometer in Uganda might not suffice to satisfy any of these assumptions. Instead of facilitating the life of an individual with diabetes, the glucometer might confuse it and, in some cases, make life even harder. After introducing the practicalities and impracticalities of how to put a glucometer to use, I will scrutinize one significant assumption about the glucometer. A claim that is indicated as a warning in many glucometer user manuals: a glucometer should not be used for the diagnosis of diabetes.

While I do not offer a detailed description of glucometer user guides here, I do aim to picture selected aspects and extracts I found in different user guides, which will be of relevance here. The glucometer hereby does not only serve as a medical technology that is used for medical purposes, but as a means through which different narratives can be conveyed and transported. Different ways of using the technology may come to the fore when a technology is transferred to a setting alien to its country of design and origin. The user manual gives us an idea about the intended use and offers us a background against which the glucometer can be translated and/or contested.

Know it, get it started and "make your life easier"

This part intends to offer some insights in the general use and application of the glucometer. How are certain aspects stated in the user guide of a glucometer translated or "tinkered" against the backdrop of (technological) scarcity in Uganda? What do actors involved do with the given information? Hereby we should keep in mind, that not every user might read the user guide in the first place. In many of the health facilities I have visited in Uganda, the manual was absent. Or the glucometer was delivered without the manual. Further we should acknowledge the fact that there is never something like an "ordinary" user of technology.

Only by briefly skimming through different user guides that come with glucometers, it becomes clear quite fast that there are a few aspects we ought to know and should consider before we start using the device. If we do not follow the guidelines, we are cautioned, the meter may not function properly, give wrong testing results or even break. Many glucometer companies lure their customers with the "easy use" and the simple, accurate way to test whole blood glucose (sugar) levels, anytime and anywhere. The at times 88-pages long user manuals, through which we have to maneuver before getting the glucometer started, seem to contradict this promise. 88 pages with different features of what the technology has to offer and warnings, which of these features may no longer function if we use the device differently. I will assess descriptions and aspects that can be found in glucometer user manuals, informing us about its intended functions and use. Further I will take a closer look at one very specific warning stated in nearly all the manuals: the glucometer is not to be used for the diagnosis of diabetes.

All the user guides I have considered here derive from glucometers brands I found to be used in different health facilities in Uganda. The National Medical Stores (NMS) is the responsible body for the procurement and distribution of medicines and other medical equipment to governmental health centers. Though it is said that the NMS only cater for one brand and type of glucometer, I counted at least 18 different brands and types of glucometers that were used (or not usable) in health facilities, though they were not on the procurement list. Glucometers with names like Accu Chek, Accu Chek Active, Accu Chek Aviva, Freestyle Optium Xceed, Freestyle Optium, Soft Style or TRUEresult, just to name a few. Though they differ in types and brands, the user manuals show some commonalities: when we open the user guide, firstly we are welcomed, thanked for and congratulated to the successful purchase of the glucometer. We are assured that we have made the best deal imaginable. For example: "Thank you for choosing the SD CodeFreeTM Blood Glucose Monitoring System. Your new SD CodeFreeTM Blood Glucose Monitoring System is an important tool that can help you better manage your diabetes" (Cover CodeFreeTM). Or, "Welcome to Accuracy and Convenience. [...]. We're proud to be your partner in helping you manage your diabetes" (ContourTS). These are some of the phrases through which we may get the feeling that we have made a good deal in buying exactly this type of glucometer. Words such as "Accuracy", "Convenience" and "Partner" do not make us feel like individuals who have to monitor their blood glucose levels on a regular basis because we have diabetes. We rather feel like a person in charge of the situation, a business partner.

While there clearly are visual and technical differences between the glucometers, the overall function, as mentioned, is the same for all glucometers: the measuring of the blood glucose. Most user manuals display pictures of the glucometer, which indicate descriptions and visualizations of the different functions the meter offers. In addition, they picture how to use it technically: how and where to switch the device on for testing and off after testing; where and how to insert the glucose testing strip, for the blood has to be applied to a specific spot on a glucose strip and so on. Every glucometer has a front side with a display, a glucose strip port, and some devices also have a glucose strip release button (otherwise the strip is simply pulled out manually without a button). The backside of the glucometer has a battery door for inserting a battery, a coin cell in most of the cases. Further every glucometer has a serial number, which is the identification number of the device, alongside a phone number that can be called for assistance if required.[3]

When we use the glucometer for the first time we have to make sure that we have inserted the battery correctly, different symbols may appear on the screen such as a temperature symbol either indicating the temperature (if the temperature of the testing environment is too high or too low), a drop symbol that tells us when to apply blood and confirms whether or not enough blood has been applied, a battery symbol that lets us know when we should buy a new battery. In fact, coin cells are not only expensive but also hardly available especially in the rural areas of Uganda and therefore one of the reasons for non-useable glucometers.

We are further informed that the glucose testing strips should not be used either after their expiration date, which is indicated on the testing strip vial, and we should not use the strips longer than three months after we have opened the vial. We are advised to write the date of opening onto the vial, to stay within the time frame. If we use the testing strips after the expiration or past the three months after opening, we may receive incorrect testing results. In this case, we are advised to discard the testing strips and replace them by new testing strips.

The manual states the importance of blood glucose monitoring with a glucometer and that the more knowledgeable we are about diabetes in general, the better we will be able to take care of our health. Together with our doctor or a diabetes health care specialist we should discuss the frequency of testing as well as our individual target ranges for our blood glucose results. The closer we get to our target range, respectively if most of the tests we perform are within the target range, we can assume that our treatment plan is well adjusted and the diabetes is well controlled. This in turn will prevent complications, which might occur in the course of the disease.[4] Understanding the glucose levels requires that the numbers and the way they are displayed on the glucometer are correctly understood. There are two different units of measuring the blood sugar: mg/dL and mmol/l. There is a way of translating mg/dL into mmol/l by dividing the digits by the factor of 18. Vice versa it is possible to convert mmol/l into mg/dL by multiplying the result with the factor of 18.[5] Both units are different labels for the same measured variable,

---

[3] In fact, I tried to call different service numbers from Uganda and have not reached anyone on the published numbers.

[4] It is important to note that the positive effect of continuous blood-glucose monitoring for individuals with type-diabetes, who are not using insulin as treatment is strongly debated and there are hardly studies that confirm a positive effect on the treatment outcome. Individuals with type 1 diabetes as well as individuals with type 2 diabetes who are on insulin, however, are required to monitor their glucose levels regularly. Later in we will see that continuous monitoring can be especially helpful in cases where individuals live far away from the next health care center or have instable glucose levels.

[5] Example: 7 mmol/l times 18 = 126 mg/dL or 145 mg/dL divided by 18 = 8 mmI/l.

the concentration of glucose in the blood. Yet in order to understand the units of measuring, both types have to be known, for some glucometers have a preset unit, which cannot be changed: "Note: Factory set, cannot be changed by user", it simply says in one of the manuals.

While for the US context, the standard unit for measuring glucose is in mg/dL, and the glucometers produced in the US or for the US are all preset in this unit, in Uganda there is no formalized common unit. Some hospitals use mg/dL, while others use mmol/l, depending on the glucometer they are using. The different way in which the glucose levels are displayed can have consequences for the use and interpretation of the glucose levels. One health center I visited thought the glucometer was faulty and would indicate wrong results when the test results were displayed in mg/dL instead of mmol/l. Further, though there are hardly any guidelines of how to go about the testing and treatment for diabetes in Uganda, the ones that exist, such as the cut-off values for when an individual has glucose levels in the diabetes range, are stated in mmol/l and not in mg/dL.[6] "This makes work harder when it comes to comparing the results on a district level or country level", a statistician told me. "Some health centers either do not indicate levels at all or they write them in mg/dL in the documentation books. In this case I have to calculate all the levels in order to have uniformity. Even the health centers that calculate themselves, some of them make mistakes using the wrong multiplication factor. For example, 8 instead of 18, or they do not have a calculator and have calculation errors. This makes it complicated and tiresome at times and also I think there is a lot of faulty data out there", he continued.

When we go on with reading the manual the reader is constantly addressed with personal pronouns in relation to the technology and the testing: "your test results", "your target ranges", "your [gluco]meter" etc. While this makes us feel personally addressed, involved and connects us to the glucometer as "the owner" of it, this does not necessarily apply to Uganda. A glucometer is often not in the possession of one single person, but is used to test many individuals in health centers. This brings us to the next aspect. After we are familiar with the rather technical and external functions of the glucometer, there are further things we have to understand when we put a glucometer to use. Because if we do not use the glucometer as we are advised in the manual, we are warned, the ability to determine the true blood glucose levels cannot be guaranteed. We should never use a testing strip more than once, and never apply water, alcohol or any cleaner to the test strip. The reuse of test strips "will cause inaccurate results". After we have applied one drop of blood

---

6 Most individuals who were engaging in self-testing preferred to measure in mml/l because "in mg the number feels too much as they are higher than with mml. The number in mmol/l looks smaller than the mg. That makes the numbers less threatening", an individual once explained to me.

we should not apply another drop as this will indicate an error. The next information we receive, printed in capital and partly bold letters, is that the blood glucose monitoring system is "for one person use **ONLY**. **DO NOT** share your [gluco]meter [...] with anyone, including family members. **DO NOT** use on more than one person" (emphasis in the original)[7].

I have met individuals who shared a glucometer with others within a community. A type of glucometer-sharing that saves expenses in the acquirement of the device and enables to engage in self-monitoring outside of the hospital setting. If there was more than one person with diabetes within one family, it was a common practice to share a glucometer because "it is good that we can share, we can help each other with the testing and we save some money", like a woman with diabetes once said. Most importantly, in many governmental health facilities of Uganda one glucometer serves the patients of an entire hospital, in some cases several hundreds of individuals who are all being tested with one and the same glucometer. "It is possible to use one glucometer for all of them, because it is only the testing strip, which has to be changed. So every person only needs an own strip, but I use the same glucometer for all of them", a diabetes nurse explained, when she tried to make sense of the claim "do not use for more than one person".

There was some skepticism about using only one glucometer for many patients on the side of a laboratory technician working in a private laboratory in Kampala where glucometers were not used at all. He was thinking that

> "if you use it [the glucometer] for more than one person, different levels of glucose are coming together inside the meter. So there is some inbuilt level already, you add on that and you declare one being diabetic, put them on treatment, but yet you should not, because it was actually the blood from the other person you have tested before. Personally I am opposed, seriously opposed to use these glucometers. Especially when it comes to health facilities. The best we can do, I don't know how, people should get access to real machines [the bigger laboratory methods] that can do this work."

I met a medical professor at a German institute that focuses its research on glucometers. He explained, and this resonates with the descriptions in the user manuals of the glucometers, that glucometers are predominantly produced for therapy control and self-monitoring practices. That is what it is meant to do: measure glucose levels anywhere and anytime. It is this capacity, that should make the life of an individual with diabetes "easier". "Designed to make your life easier" – one of the promises the glucometer holds. "Making your life easier" with a high-quality medical device, delivering fast results. It is easy to handle and most importantly it

---

7 Taken from the TRUEresult blood glucose monitoring system user manual: http://www.niprodiagnostics.eu/suitsyou/dyn/files/trueresult-owners-booklet.pdf

is meant and made to be the everyday tool with which blood glucose can be overseen and controlled. Inevitably the question arises "easier than what?" or "easier as compared to when?" Many of the diabetes patients who own a glucometer in Uganda have only recently started using it outside of the hospital setting, if at all. By talking to some of these few patients, I started to doubt that their life was actually made easier with the glucometer. At times, even the contrary was the case as now they had "to worry about another thing", namely taking care of a medical device, which had to be kept going by purchasing expensive and at time unavailable batteries. The testing strips were expensive and at times unavailable too. And it was not at all that easy to use. In fact, it was more than once that I was told life had been easier without the glucometer. Without the glucometer, the responsibility "for life" and "for testing" was in the hands of professionals and not in the hands of one individual alone. Further it was easier simply because they "didn't have to look at the meter lying in the shelf unused because the money is not there to buy the strips or batteries", an individual explained. What was thought of making the life of an individual with diabetes easier may therefore cause the opposite in a setting like Uganda. Not only using and interpreting the test results, but continuously assuring the availability of spare parts such as strips or batteries, and the emotional pressure the glucometer may exert, when a patient sees the meter being unused.

There were also a few patients who, despite the fact that they owned a glucometer, preferred to be tested in the hospital. For some it was rather complicated to understand and interpret the numbers correctly all the time. As a patient explained "I prefer to test myself from the hospital. Okay you can test from home, but still it is risky, because you might check yourself from home and assume that you are fine, because you do not understand the numbers correctly." Many patients preferred being tested in the hospitals, sharing the responsibility for their chronic condition. Using the glucometer for the daily monitoring of the blood glucose level is often not sustainable in Uganda. Instead the glucometer is used at times when a patient feels unwell or in cases where the readings are worrying.

Nevertheless, the basic prerequisite for using the glucometer is the availability of the testing strips and batteries in the first place. Even if a glucometer is available, as soon as the strips are not, a test cannot be performed. There are other incidents, which complicate and prevent testing: If the testing strips are available, but the batteries have died (or it is hard to find the suitable battery), a test cannot be performed; if the result the glucometer indicates is displayed in a unit that is unknown, a test result cannot be understood; and if the display indicates an error, which cannot be rectified (often especially because the manuals that come with the meter are discarded right in the beginning), a glucometer will fail to do what it was allegedly meant to do right from the start.

The problem with the travel and influx of medical technology is not that it is there, but its technical compatibility. Glucometers from one brand can only be used together with the strips of the same brand and model. Meaning the good-meant presents from family members or friends buying glucometers outside of Uganda are useless as soon as the strips are finished. In most cases it is then not possible to replace them. The technology quickly becomes useless, and obsolete. In some health facilities, there were collections of unused and discarded glucometers: glucometer graveyards, devices in different colors, different sizes and meters in need of different kinds of testing strips. A technology that was designed and produced to make life easier for people with diabetes, to facilitate self-testing, was sometimes complicating life. The best technology will be of no use if it lacks the, most basic supplies.

Compared to a country like Germany, where it is easy to get a free glucometer as a promotion from one of the several companies there are, in Uganda, it is not easy or even impossible to get a free meter. In Germany, you can order the strips for your meters online, you can even place a repeat order and strips will be sent to you on a regular basis. This is not possible in Uganda. In Germany, patients are supported by their health insurance. In Uganda, hardly anybody has health insurance.[8] In Uganda patients can test themselves when they feel sick to confirm their status, in Germany part of the self-monitoring entails self-testing several times per day. But with a single strip, worth up to three dollars, this is an expensive undertaking in Uganda.

Though it is never mentioned explicitly we may assume that all this information is given on the assumption that first of all we, as the buyers or receivers of the glucometer, are literate and have purchased a meter in our home country so that we may understand the manual. In the case of Uganda, though the official language is English, not all people are able to read and understand English. But there are further obstacles: as mentioned, we have to be able to understand the units of measurement, be it mg/dL or mmol/l. And most importantly, it is assumed that we have bought the glucometer under the condition that we are able to provide for everything it will need in order to run and keep functioning (buying batteries and more glucose strips when they are finished etc.). In short: as easy as it may seem to put the glucometer to use in one setting, might not necessarily function as easily in a context like Uganda. While I have given an overview of the glucometer, its functions and which difficulties users might face in general terms, the next part

---

8   A woman I once met in Uganda working for an insurance company explained that people are grouped in different age groups. People above the age of 60 by the time they want to start a health insurance are not covered at all. The same accounts for people with type 1 diabetes. People with type 2 diabetes are usually not insured either, or if so, then with a very high premium. "It is the same when you get in a car accident and you go to the insurance the next day and expect them to pay. That is not possible, we also have to earn our shillings", the woman explained. It is different when an individual is working for a company or an organization that offers cooperate insurance, in this case they also cover both types of diabetes.

will focus on one of the core purposes of the glucometer in Uganda, the diagnosis of diabetes. Thereby, it shows that the glucometer is not as unproblematically applicable as a diagnostic tool as it may seem.

Not for diagnosis?

Medical technologies are usually understood as devices that bring to the fore what would not be possible, visible or quantifiable without them. Some medical devices are able to roentgenize our body and search for broken bones like an X-Ray. Others are able to measure our heartbeats with an ultrasound heart scan. Again others, like the microscope, can see things in our blood that the human eye cannot, like parasites. Or, as in the case of the glucometer, measure the amount of sugar in the blood. A medical device is able to facilitate a diagnosis, and can assist us in making the invisible (within our body) visible (on a display). The test results are communicated differently. They may be designated as a color (e.g. blue is negative, pink is positive), as a graphic display (two bars typify a positive, one bar typifies a negative result), or as a number that represents the amount of glucose in our blood and has to be categorized ultimately. Medical technologies share the alleged commonality that they (should) facilitate a diagnosis, or that they are the basic means to approach and establish a diagnosis. While the next chapter will take a closer look at the moment of diagnosis and the role technology plays in diagnosing in Uganda, for the following I suggest to understand technologies simply as tools that can do – or assist us in doing – what we as human beings could not do without them. As a matter of fact, there are few medical devices that are not made to assist in establishing a diagnosis. Diagnosing is what most point-of-care devices are meant to do.

While we were able to read in the user guide what the glucometer can allegedly do – above all measure the glucose in one's blood – we are also informed, or rather warned what it cannot do, namely do exactly what it is expected to do: diagnose. As written in a user guide, the glucometer "should be used only for testing purposes [...]. It should not be used for the diagnosis of diabetes."[9] But what if there is only this one means to uncover diabetes? What else can be done in a context like Uganda, where, as mentioned before, the glucometer is often the first- and often

---

9 In one manual I read, there was no explicit mention that the glucometer should not be used for the diagnosis of diabetes. It simply stated that the glucometers intended use is for self-monitoring practices. I contacted some glucometer companies – by using the customer service indicated in the manuals – to inquire an explanation as to why a glucometer is not suitable for diagnoses. I sought an answer and assessment from the companies who produce these technologies. But the only answer I received was that "a glucometer is not intended to diagnose but is a technology that facilitates self-monitoring."

only-choice technology when it comes to the diagnosis of diabetes? It is then not a matter of choice whether or not the glucometer can be used for this purpose. But it is simply the only tool available in order to uncover and as a result treat and manage diabetes. There is no other choice than translate this claim into a claim that is applicable to the setting to which it is applied. While this warning hints at a difference between testing and diagnosing[10], it is another aspect we will look at: the translation and molding of a technology, which, at least in some governmental health facilities in Uganda, does what it is allegedly not supposed to do. Or, to put it differently: the glucometer, which is *not used* for diagnosis in the minority world, *is used* for diagnosis in Uganda.

The translation of technology, especially if it is related to disease, respectively the diagnosis of a disease, might come with a risk. In the case of the glucometer it is the risk of false diagnoses. Unfortunately, I was not able to meet with any designers or creators of glucometers, but as mentioned before, I was able to meet a professor from a German university. He has been dealing with and conducting research on glucometers for the past years, testing different types and brands of glucometers in terms of quality, accuracy, price, functions and its handling. He told me that though there were a few devices with a relatively good measurement accuracy, studies, which confirm that a glucometer can be used for diagnostic purposes unhesitatingly, are still lacking. The glucometers' sensitivity to moisture and temperature for instance, or the storage conditions are factors that could have an influence on the accuracy of the testing results, "heat and moisture are most likely a problem in Uganda, too, as it is close to the equator", he reasoned. A medical doctor from a governmental health facility added the following to this point:

> "How sure can you be that a glucometer gives the right result? And if you use a strip, how sure are you the strip is ok? Storage is so important. One of the most important aspects of a laboratory is storage. Uganda is in the tropics. Many things come from abroad where the temperature is much lower. Most of the kits are manufactured in those low temperatures. But at times you will find testing taking place in the sun like this, where the glucometer is placed on a bench in the sun. When you go to the field in the villages it is even worse. There you have 30 degrees Celsius and they should be on 10. We might tell people they are diabetic, when they are not or tell them they are fine, when they are not because of our methodology. It is a challenge."

To find out whether a glucometer is giving accurate or nearly accurate results is firstly possible if the results it produces are compared to the results of bigger lab-

---

10 In Luganda, the language commonly spoken in the central region of Uganda, there is no difference made between testing and diagnosis. Both, diagnosis as well as testing would be translated with Okukebela Sukali, which means check or test the sugar.

oratory machinery. Other laboratory methods for the diagnosis of diabetes are, however, hardly available in most governmental health facilities. "Some glucometers are better than others", the German professor explained, "and this is not necessarily price-dependent. It is therefore impossible to assess the quality of the meter, without any control tests". Unless the glucometer has for instance fallen down and is obviously broken or the testing strips are cracked or bent, it is not possible to see whether or not it functions properly and gives accurate results. In Germany for instance, diagnoses are not established with capillary blood (blood from the fingertip, as it is the case when you test with a glucometer), exactly because of this reason. Instead, to confirm the presence of diabetes other methods are applied, which use venous blood from the crook of the arm. The difference between the results of a measurement with a glucometer as compared to the measurement with a laboratory method can diverge up to 25% (Baumstark et al. 2017). There can be great deviations if there is a misalignment. The medical professor and his team once tested a glucometer with such a misalignment and concluded that if it would have been used for diagnostic purposes, one quarter of the tests would have been false positive diagnoses. However,

> "if the results are 11 mmol/l or more it is relatively obvious that an individual has diabetes because it is high. But it is the borderline values where such a misalignment can have enormous negative effects. If an individual has a glucose level of 6,7 mmol/l it is not so obvious whether a patient has diabetes or not. With a misalignment and the normal deviation of 20% it is possible that the patient either has 5,5 mmol/l or 7,8 mmol/l. Both is possible and decisive whether or not an individual has diabetes or not. With 5,5 clearly not, with 7,8 clearly yes. Further the values of capillary blood are generally higher than venous blood."[11]

Factors such as whether or not an individual has eaten before the testing have an additional influence on the test result. An individual who has eaten, can easily achieve a glucose level of 8,9 mmol/l and more, though being completely healthy, a value that actually indicates diabetes. Without the reassurance whether or not she or he has eaten, a healthy individual might leave a doctor's office or laboratory as a patient diagnosed with diabetes. Not only the accuracy of the machine influences the result, but also the way it is used. The alleged simplicity of the device may obscure the far-reaching effects it can have when not using it properly: this includes simple, pre-analytical aspects, such as having clean fingers before the testing (if you have eaten a banana and test without washing your fingers, your results will

---

11 Before the development of other laboratory methods, capillary blood was used for diagnosis in Germany, too. But due to the vast differences between the test results, the glucometer was soon discharged as a diagnostic tool.

4. A 'simple' technology and its translations: the glucometer

be high); quick testing (not waiting too long until the blood is inserted into the strip) and that the testing strips themselves are handled with care.

The biggest problem though, is that it is not visible from the outside if a glucometer is faulty, has a bad quality, or whether the control strips are of good quality and give relatively accurate results. Yet there is a possibility to assess whether or not the device is functioning without contrasting the results to other testing results[12]. Every glucometer comes with a control solution, which, in theory, should be used when a glucometer is put to use for the first time, every time a new glucose strip tin is opened or the battery has been changed, or in case the individual feels the results of the test are deviating extremely from the way she or he feels. For instance, the device shows a very high glucose level, but from the symptoms the individual has, it rather feels like having low glucose levels.

However, the control solution was not used in the governmental facilities I visited, but rather discarded immediately. If I found control solutions in the storages of the laboratories, they had often expired or were not kept in the fridge, as recommended. "Do you think anyone uses the control solution?", I was once rhetorically asked by a laboratorian from a private laboratory that did not use glucometers for the diagnosis of diabetes. He answered his own question by stating

> "They don't! They throw the control solution away. So sooner or later they will start going blind, because they do not check the glucometer as recommended. The control solution is something that gives you a direction. It checks you, the user, it checks the machine, it checks the reagent, in this case the strip. So if you don't have a control or calibrator you are going blind, just producing results blindly and this might be dangerous for the people who are tested."

The German professor confirmed that this also the case for many German health facilities: "using the control solution is nothing anybody does" (see also Johnson et al. 2017). Though in Germany the guidelines require to use the control solution once a day when a glucometer[13] is applied in a doctor's office, it is rarely done. Because firstly, the control solution is only an approximate indication. And secondly, it has to be stored properly in a fridge. When the control solution is used, however, it has to have room temperature, which makes the procedure more complicated and tiresome. Not to mention that fridges are not necessarily found or fully functional in governmental health facilities in Uganda.

---

12 I have met individuals with diabetes who owned more than one glucometer and were able to contrast the results of the testing among the different devices. But this is not only a costly practice, it is also very rare.
13 Please note that the glucometers used in German doctor's offices are not the same ones as used for self-monitoring practices. They are more expensive devices that are specifically produced for doctor's offices.

Despite the factors mentioned thus far, the uncertainty whether or not the glucometer functions and gives accurate results, the glucometer still remains the only means in many places in Uganda to diagnose diabetes. When I confronted some of the individuals with this claim, that glucometers should not be used for the diagnosis of diabetes, I encountered different ways of how people made sense of this statement. One of the individuals I met, 27-year-old Samuel who, unlike many other individuals with diabetes in Uganda, himself owned a glucometer, too, stumbled over this information. His explanation for why this warning is indicated in the user's guide was not related to the mere possibility of the device giving inaccurate results, but focused on the responsibility and expertise of medical professionals in making diagnoses:

> "There is this warning, that it [the glucometer] is not supposed to be used for diagnosis, it is for home use. But I know what this means. They [the producers] are telling us because we might rule out. We are not medical personnel, we can end up ruling out things, which are not true. They were meaning if you are not medical personnel, don't use it. Because you might think... Listen... digits of a diabetic person differ from one who is normal. Now, already if you have a glucometer for home use means that you are diabetic, and you know the numbers you are supposed to follow, which don't apply for a normal person. When they say home use, it is for home use, for you who is diabetic. Now being diabetic and buying a glucometer doesn't make you a doctor. So it doesn't mean that when your wife or your husband starts telling you, I feel headache, my eyes, I cannot see well... then you diagnose and say go and get metformin [a pharmaceutical for the treatment of diabetes that lowers the blood sugar levels]. Anybody can buy the glucometer. It does not mean that a random person goes and buys a glucometer and can diagnose anybody without consulting a doctor."

A biomedical engineer and a laboratory technician working for a company that has been selling and distributing medical and laboratory equipment to private health facilities in Uganda since the 1960s reasoned in a discussion amongst each other:

> **Biomedical Engineer:** "For me I think it [the statement that the glucometer should not be used for the diagnosis of diabetes] means that not everybody can make a diagnosis. I give you an example, for making an ultrasound there are technicians who take an image of you. But it is not the technician who will diagnose. It is not him who will tell you what's wrong with you."
>
> **Laboratory Technician:** "What he is saying is true, because what it could mean is that the glucometer gives you results. It just gives you results. But someone with higher profession has to diagnose the label what is wrong with you. That's what it means, I think. He was trying to give you an example with a scan or an image. They are technicians and will take the picture and tell you, you have

a broken bone but he will not write the report. You get the point? He will then give it to the radiologist who will tell you your bone is broken at this degree angle."

Biomedical Engineer: "For diabetes, it is the clinician who does the diagnosis. Because the symptoms are referring to a disease and probably its cause also. With the glucometer, anyone can have it. Like I can go and buy it and I have no real idea, not even of the procedure. When it is this number, it means this. Or if it is negative. That's not a diagnosis, but its only testing."

Indeed, why should a glucometer, the only available technology in Uganda for the diagnosis of diabetes should not be used if it was a medical professional using it? A laboratory technician working in a private lab, where they were not using glucometers but perform blood analyses for the diagnosis of diabetes, had also not heard about this before. Or as he put it: "So what is it [the glucometer] for if it is not for diagnosis?" He was wondering why it was permitted to use a technology for a purpose that it was not designed for. In his eyes, it was the responsibility of the Ministry of Health of Uganda to take care that every individual in Uganda received the best care and treatment there was. "And if we are not giving them the best because we think it is too expensive, then we are killing them earlier than they should have died", he continued. We were wondering, if it was ultimately better to use the glucometer to diagnose diabetes than to not diagnose it at all? Was the awareness of the potential errors and inaccuracy of the glucometer a reason not to use it? Another laboratory technician, however, concluded that

> "it is not ok to use the machine. We might think it is cheap but at times it is turning our lives upside down and it is costing our lives. People are going to die because we misdiagnose them with a technology that is not made for this purpose. In most health facilities, you will find the same machine they used two or three years ago. That cannot be true. Even a car you have to service. Every machine has to be serviced. As I told you earlier you are not sure whether what you are giving is right because you do not have any measures that are put in place to know if yesterday the machine was right, what makes you think the machine is right today? How sure can you be that after one year the machine, which has not been serviced because there is nothing like servicing it, is still working? If you are looking at an estimate, it is fine. If you are looking for an accurate diagnosis for research then it is not fine, because the result will vary from meter to meter. But as an estimate, as an epidemiological tool everyone has now agreed on that you can use a glucometer."

Point-of-care devices do not only promise convenience, but most of them are exactly made to diagnose disease. Think of RDTs, the Rapid Diagnostic Test for the diagnosis of malaria or the HIV quick test to diagnose HIV, both are tests, with which a result "positive" or "negative" result can be received within 20 minutes. The glucometer is in no way inferior concerning its use and the quickness of the testing results. "But what is it for if not for diagnosis" hints at the perception and expectation towards a medical device. A medical device that produces a result is meant for diagnosing.

What is characteristic for the use the glucometer is that it is used for both, the diagnosis as well as the monitoring of diabetes. It draws its importance from the diagnosis that happens prior to its application of continuous testing. When an individual starts to use a glucometer for self-monitoring purposes, a diagnosis has usually already been established and the doctor has informed the patient that it is useful to purchase a glucometer in order to engage in self-monitoring practices. The test seems so easy: the glucometer will indicate a number, which is displayed on a small monitor and carries the image of its correct calculation. On the contrary, it can be completely wrong, without the user recognizing or knowing it. The glucometer freely moves across Uganda or comes to Uganda from other countries without hindrances, as it seems. You may find hospitals where there are several meters, which are not in use any more and you will find medical staff who is using this technology to diagnose diabetes. The glucometer thus does both in Uganda, it diagnoses (where it can) and it sometimes does not diagnose (where it cannot or where it is not available).

I examined one of the main statements that can be found in many user manuals, namely that the glucometer is not meant to be used for the diagnosis of diabetes. I have highlighted some of the core problems for why its use for diagnostic purposes can be contested and considered to be problematic or even dangerous. Yet I did not intend to pinpoint any medical misconduct when using the glucometer to make a diagnosis of diabetes in Uganda. However, I did want to shed light on the fact that the circumstances and especially the technology involved for the diagnosis of diabetes should not simply be taken for granted or remain unquestioned. The results the device produces can of course be accurate. But it is equally possible that they are wrong without the users necessarily recognizing the results as in fact being wrong. As simple as the glucometer respectively its application seems to be, its use may have major implications for its users, the patients, as well as the larger health care system in Uganda. We may eventually come to question the technology and wonder what it actually renders visible. The following section will discuss these findings and suggest that, at the end of the day, care for diabetes is highly dependent on keeping testing going. There is more to it apart from what the glucometer allegedly can do or not do.

Keeping the testing going

The global market offers a profusion of different glucometers. There are slight differences between these medical devices in terms of look and in some functions. Yet they all have been designed to quantify the blood glucose of individuals with diabetes. The producers in the minority world battle each other with new functions, new designs, better and easier handling, cheaper models etc. In Uganda access to this great variety of glucometers is restricted. Instead, health centers and individuals have to take what is available. What does this restricted access and availability of this medical technology mean for individuals with diabetes who need it? And further, to recall the research question of this book once again, what does it mean for the visibility of diabetes in Uganda's health care system and beyond?

Medical technologies are made to facilitate care or make care possible in the first place. This chapter has shown, that despite the fact that there is an allegedly easy to use technology, there are conditions in which this easy use is complicated by structural circumstances. A medical device like the glucometer does not function on its own, it has to be operated and put to work and it has to be maintained and cared for in order for it to continue operating (Mol 2000). Moreover, it is important to understand why a device is doing what it is doing, or has stopped to do what it was purportedly meant to do. If the essential supplies, such as batteries or the glucose testing strips are lacking, then even the highest standard and up-to-date technology will fail to fulfill its duty. A technology, especially a medical device, holds a promise. The promise to improve a physical condition and its care, which is more uncertain and unstable without it – and it holds the promise of delivering a correct result and therefore suggests objectivity (Nelkin and Tancredi 1994).

I have analyzed different statements made about the glucometer, which were indicated in different user manuals. Though claimed to be, the glucometer at the end of the day is not at all that simple as the user guide promises it to be. When using it in a different way than indicated in the manual, it may give wrong results or break. There is a discrepancy between an (available) technology, which is easy to use so that it can be used in self-care and the far-reaching effect it might have, such as false diagnoses, if it is not used as the product designer has had it in mind. We were able to see that none of these statements or practices inscribed into the technological device are as straightforward in Uganda: testing strips are used after expiration date, testing results displayed in unknown measuring units are misunderstood and may cause confusion. One single glucometer, which is not meant to be used for more than one person is used for and shared between different people of an entire health facility. If an individual privately owns a glucometer, she or he will most likely share the meter with others in the family or community. This does not only have financial benefits as the costs for buying the device, the testing strips and the battery are shared, it benefits a greater number of individuals in need of the device who could not afford it on their own. The glucometer, which was meant to be a one-person-technology transforms into a device that caters for all those in need of it. It becomes a multi-person-technology. The device, which promises "to make life easier" does not make the life of an individual easier if the structural circumstances do not apply to its working. For economically deprived settings and individuals often lacking knowledge about diabetes, this is a serious challenge.

Finally, while designed for self-monitoring, conditions of scarcity transform the glucometer into a technology that is the first and at times only means to establish diagnoses of diabetes. This in turn has an influence on how the glucometer is understood in Uganda: it is hard to access it and therefore ever so valuable as it cannot be easily replaced. How do we perceive care if the choices we have to care for people are limited? All this shows that bringing a glucometer to Uganda is not a mere act of technology transfer and implementation. It rather needs to be actively adapted to and translated into a new setting. In this case, it is the act of translating the glucometer that helps to make life and care practices easier and keeps diabetes care going, and not the technology itself. Without a translation of the device, care for diabetes would not or only hardly be possible, especially in governmental health facilities.

The increased number of people with diabetes, calls for an adaptation of healthcare systems who are often not well prepared to deal with the high burden of these conditions economically, politically, and technologically. However, especially diabetes is a disease that comes into being and that is enacted through technology, as the next chapter will picture. Without testing, there will be no diabetes, or rather no scientifically confirmed case of diabetes, not on paper and not in any records. Testing, respectively diagnosing, is an essential aspect of the classification of disease. Not the translation alone, but also the prospect of using a technological device in the first place comes with benefits. Further it is not enough to put a technological device, like the glucometer, to use. The device will do something, it will create something. First and foremost, it is a number the device produces, but it is even more than that as chapter six intends to depict. Furthermore, I examined the very conditions, in which this technology is translated differently, produces different results or treatment, or in other words, the conditions in which it evolves and comes into being. Focusing on the practices and explanations of people in the field, I proved the glucometers fluidity as it travels the globe.

We should also think about existing technological possibilities, especially today, where technology seems to be ubiquitous and seems to be able to manage almost anything, any disease, any condition. Why does that matter? It matters because a lack of choices necessarily will lead to a lack of possibilities and ways to manage a disease. It influences the way, in which the device can but also has to be translated and what is made visible accordingly. On the rear, as we have seen, and as Annemarie Mol has shown for diabetes in the Netherlands, more choices (e.g. in our case more brands and types of glucometers) will not necessarily lead to better treatment and disease management (Mol 2008). Certainly, it seems that good diabetes management is a matter of care and not merely technology. A matter of care that may play out differently in Uganda and the Netherlands, but still certainly is a matter of care. As I suggested, the translation of the glucometer from global markets to its various application contexts in Uganda show that, analytically, we need to bring the study of translation together with studying care. In order to account for the differences that translations produce, we need to study how people care for, struggle to care for, or indeed are unable to care for the translated technological device and the people it is meant to serve. A successfully translated, fluid technology requires care, it is not only a matter of selling the device or making it available, but entails efforts in finding new ways of creative adaptation.

The glucometer has the freedom to travel within a country and from other countries without hindrances, you may find hospitals where there are several meters, which are not in use any more. You will equally find those that are using this technology to diagnose diabetes. Those are aspects that the global markets surely do not take into consideration when they produce glucometers. In the case of impoverished health systems what they were thought to be used for in the beginning ends up being shifted from homes to the labs and beyond. Chronic diseases have common features concerning the level and need of care, the level of medical involvement and also the personal lives, anxieties, hopes and whatever there might be. Being diagnosed with a chronic condition entails the certainty that life is uncertain and that it will never be the way it used to be. Going to the health center regularly, taking medication, having to be tested over again to test the status. Ups and downs, moments of healthiness, moments of illness and moments of despair. Here a diagnostic device, instead of alleviating the uncertainties, may contribute to new uncertainties. In Uganda and elsewhere, the glucometer does not only mean the entry point into a life with disease, but also the entry point to a life characterized by uncertainty and a life in need of (medical) care. But it is in countries like Uganda, where the only possibilities to be diagnosed with diabetes is through the access to and the availability of the glucometer.

This chapter gave an overview of the practicalities surrounding the glucometer, the main actor of this book. In the next chapter, the diagnosis of diabetes shall be the focus of inquiry. Hereby you will get to know individuals and their quest for a diagnosis and meet caregivers who establish diabetes diagnoses. We will enter different diagnostic spaces in governmental as well as private health facilitates; and we will realize that there is not necessarily a big difference whether or not an individual can access private or governmental services that determines a diagnosis of diabetes. Suffice to say that it is also not only a matter of access to and the availability of technology whether or not a diagnosis can be made in Uganda, but also a matter of chance.

5. Diagnostic detours and a logic of chance

> Our lives unfold in ways that surprise us, that force us to recognize the uncertainty of things. We live, by and large, with no clear recognition of how things will end, trying to portend the significance of current events in light of a future we can only imagine —Mattingly and Garro 2000: 184.

When we fall ill, or we suspect to be ill, we will most certainly sooner or later search for a reason for our symptoms. We might wonder about the most likely cause for, and try different remedies against our ailments even before we consult a doctor. Perhaps we will ask our family or friends for advice, consult books or check the internet to find answers. Yet when we feel threatened by these inscrutable symptoms, or when they persist over a period of time and do not dissolve with the measures we have taken (e.g. take painkillers, take a rest etc.), we will in all likelihood at some point find ourselves in a doctor's office for further consultation. As Mol and her colleagues note, the reason for why people seek care in the first place is because "their bodies happen to not submit to their wishes, let alone their commands", the bodies have become unruly and uncontrollable (Mol, Moser and Pols 2010: 10). On the one hand, it will be our goal to find ways to get rid of the nasty symptoms that fill our thoughts with fear and uncertainty if something bigger, even life-threatening might stand for and behind these symptoms. On the other hand, it is an answer to our ailments we are after, the certainty of what was and is paining us. Especially when the symptoms persist over a long period of time or when the answers we have received were unsatisfying or seemed to be wrong. It is then that we want to hear a name, a term, a designation and an explanation for these symptoms: it is a diagnosis we seek (Jutel 2011; Balint 1964/2002).[1] It is, however, equally possible that it is exactly the answer we fear.

---

[1] Later in this book, in chapter seven, we will take a look at screening practices, where it is not the individual who initially seeks care induced by plaguing symptoms. Instead it is part of intervention strategies to uncover disease based on the assumption that the earlier a disease is diagnosed, the better the prospect of preventing severe damages of the body due to late diagnosis.

If we take a look at how the term diagnosis is defined in a common dictionary like the Merriam Webster Dictionary, diagnosis is the "a) art or act of identifying disease from its signs and symptoms [and that it is further] b) the decision reached by diagnosis". Another definition describes diagnosis as the "investigation of analysis of the cause or nature of a condition, situation, or problem [and as] a statement or conclusion from such an analysis."[2] According to these definitions diagnosis can be seen as both, the process of identifying and uncovering disease, but also as an outcome, the result and conclusion emerging from this process. It is "a vehicle for sense making [when] [t]hings that happen to the body are put into perspective" (Warren and Manderson 2016: 141).

As diagnosis is among the first responses to suffering, the moment of diagnosis as well as the diagnostic process itself are essential in the interaction between an individual and medical personnel and the technologies involved that assist them (Smith-Morris 2015: 1). It is the moment, when a doctor reaches a conclusion after weighing symptoms against different possibilities and probabilities of disease. Jutel describes the fluid nature of diagnoses referring to the work of Mirowsky and Ross (1989) who compare diagnoses to the constellations of the stars in the sky. Meaning arises from the way in which we assemble and order the stars into patterns that are recognizable and understandable for us. In fact, which symptoms we will see and find worth investigating, and which ones we will repudiate as unimportant and trivial, is highly influenced by a complex interplay of social, political, economic and technological factors. This counts for individuals with a medical as well with a non-medical background (Jutel 2011: 61).

It is worth taking a quick look at the distinction commonly made in medical anthropology (and the social sciences in general) between illness and disease as it is significant to the study of diagnosis. It involves essential conceptual differences that inform discussions of and views on diagnosis. Identifying disease includes a transformation process, which alters individually experienced illness into an objectively acknowledged disease, established with scientifically approved methods and technologies. Diagnosis is what brings perceived illness and established diagnosis together and makes them congruent in the ideal case. Kleinman distinguishes between disease and illness whereby disease is a condition of ill-health diagnosed by a doctor and illness can be understood as subjectively experienced suffering. He ascertains that "*[d]isease* refers to a malfunctioning of biological and/or psychological processes, while the term *illness* refers to the psychosocial experience and meaning of perceived disease" (Kleinman 1980: 72, emphasis in the original; cf. Mechanic 1962 and Cassell et al. 1976). Or, as Eisenberg put it, a "patient suffers 'illnesses'; doctors diagnose and treat 'disease'" (Eisenberg 1977: 9). Being ill relates to psychosocial and cultural experiences of a person, who does not only search for cure

---

[2] https://www.merriam-webster.com/dictionary/diagnosis.

but also for an explanation and a reason for being sick. By distinguishing diseases as biomedically classifiable constructs and illnesses as subjective perceptions, it becomes clear that disease and illness can also exist independently of one another. Illness can be felt without a disease being diagnosed.[3] Likewise a disease can be diagnosed, without an individual feeling ill, as we will see later.

It is the diagnostic process and the final medical conclusion emerging from this process, which brings both, illness and disease, together or attempts to do so. As we will see, at an early stage of diabetes, individuals usually do not feel much pain or experience the typical initial symptoms of diabetes as evidence of disease even though it is already present. This in turn hampers early diagnoses and delays the initiation of care, as some diseases are easier to detect than others. Easier mostly when the symptoms are allegedly obvious and leave little space for other options and possibilities. Harder when the symptoms are not clear-cut, when there are many options what the underlying disease could be, like in diabetes. Another possibility is that the symptoms are alien and unfamiliar and do not relate to anything that either the individual with these symptoms or the medical personnel in duty has heard of or experienced before. A diagnosis requires knowledge, an array of experiences and a pool of disease classification tools to connect the symptoms to a possible underlying cause. It usually requires a medically authorized person to define who is affected by a disease and by which one. Moreover, as individuals who experience unexplained symptoms, we expect and hope for "the explanatory power of the diagnosis the doctor is authorized to deliver" (Jutel 2011: 63). The difficulty of diagnosing is not only the use of knowledge and experience to identify and interpret symptoms, but also the utilization of technology when applicable.

The technology available today has generally made diagnoses and the handling of disease easier. Technology is the vehicle with which we reach our goal alongside the knowledge of when to apply it and how to use it correctly (at what time, in which place and under which conditions). But as mentioned before, some diseases (especially chronic conditions) "involve more guesswork about invisible processes and events, or about potential future events" (Smith-Morris 2016: 5). Technology in shape of a diagnostic device functions as the mediator and conveyer between the doctor or medical personnel and the individual and this is because "[t]echnology

---

3 Allan Young (1981) added an additional, social dimension to the differentiation of disease and illness with the term sickness, whereby sickness is "redefined as the process through which worrisome behavioral and biological signs, particularly ones originating in disease, are given socially recognizable meanings, i.e. they are made into symptoms and socially significant outcomes. Every culture has rules for translating signs into symptoms, for linking symptomatologies to etiologies and interventions, and for using the evidence provided by interventions to confirm translations and legitimize outcomes. The path a person follows from translation to socially significant outcome constitutes his sickness. Sickness is, then, a processor socializing disease and illness" (Young 1981: 270).

establishes, monitors, recognizes, and treats diseases" all alike (Jutel 2011: 118). It helps us to understand aspects of our body and health, which we would not be able to grasp or see without it. It has changed the way we think as human beings, how we approach health and disease but also the way in which we are able to handle it. Experiencing disease is therefore always also a technological experience.

The diagnosis of a chronic disease has far reaching implications for the lives of individuals who are diagnosed with disease. Diagnosis here is the entry point into a life that includes an imperative to act and behave in a certain way. In the case of diabetes this is for instance to omit certain foods and drinks, but also to engage in self-care. How Jutel and Dew put it "diagnosing and providing a treatment plan is only the start of what can be a messy process" (Jutel and Dew 2014: 2). The diagnostic moment is in itself an order-making tool while it at the same time creates dis-order and chaos in the lives of the (newly) diagnosed. While a diagnosis may have the character of bringing clarity and deleting diagnostic uncertainty, it may as well be the producer of it and cause anxiety and confusion. In chronic diseases, the diagnostic testing is not the end of the medical and technological encounter, but instead it is the beginning. The label 'diabetes' entails a life characterized by continuous testing. This makes it all the more important that diagnostic technology is made available and stays available.

This chapter intends to place diagnosis and testing of diabetes at the center of our attention against the backdrop of uncovering a disease with unfamiliar symptoms and often lacking technology. Since the diagnosis of diabetes is not a sudden event, but is preceded by a time of symptoms and followed by a time of medical treatment and regular blood glucose monitoring, the period before as well as after a diagnosis is equally important. Neither the approach towards nor the response to chronic disease is uniform. As much as one individual may be relieved when being diagnosed with diabetes (after a medical odyssey of searching for an answer of which disease is plaguing her or him) another individual might see her- or himself to be doomed to die.

We will see that the location in which a diagnosis is obtained can diverge: it may be a governmental health facility where services are (meant to be) free or a private clinic, where individuals will have to come up for the fees of testing, treatment and medical consultation by themselves. The person who diagnoses may be a doctor or a laboratory technician.[4] What ties all these aspects together is the matter of access and opportunity of translating a diagnosis not into a devastating labelling of one's life, but into a situation that is and remains bearable. That we rely on technology, mirrors our impuissance. At the same time, however, it is exactly this aspect, the

---

4 In chapter seven we will see that this is not necessarily the case. Instead it seems that whoever's hand holds the glucometer is allegedly able to diagnose diabetes, independent of the professional background and experience.

reliance and dependency on technology, that opens up the space and chance for using the technology in diverse ways.

As suggested in the previous chapter, I will continue to think the translations of the glucometer together with aspects of care. Diagnosis can hereby be understood as an active way of translating bodily symptoms into disease. Technology is the motor and means of translation, (the initiation of) care is the outcome thereafter. In case of diabetes, care is inherently connected to technology. Not only, because it is the technology, the glucometer, that uncovers diabetes and therefore initiates care. But especially because technology plays a decisive role in the self-care practices of individuals who will start to live lives characterized by continuous testing. The outcomes of this testing will be the basis for the steps taken in care.

Proceeding from the question of what good care is and what it entails, Annemarie Mol (2008) has offered us a useful piece to think with in her book on care, where she develops two different logics, which she juxtaposes in the course of her treatise: the logic of care and the logic of choice. The logic of care deals with the diseased body and all the activities and (human and non-human) actors involved that take care of this body, aiming to make life more bearable for a person and "actively improv[e] life" (Mol 2008: 108). As Mol and her colleagues state, "care seeks to lighten what is heavy, and even if it fails it keeps on trying". Good care is the "persistent tinkering in a world full of complex ambivalence and shifting tensions (Mol, Moser and Pols 2010: 14). It is a calm, persistent but also forgiving effort to improve a patients' situation in order to avoid deterioration. Instead of forcefully seeking for possibilities, care begins with what patients need and not what they want or know (Mol 2008: 20f). The logic of choice on the contrary can be understood as a disciplining technique that makes us individuals long for more and more choices, giving us the impression that we are capable of deciding and choosing, which type of care is best for us. The logic of choice promises us that wherever we decide to go, there will be a technology that is able to take us there. However, technologies have unexpected and sometimes undesired effects, they may generate pleasure and satisfaction, but it is equally possible that they create more suffering and uncertainty, which nobody can predict, especially when they are not available (Mol 2008: 46).

Whereas in the logic of choice the industry alongside all its advertisements promises freedom, chronic diseases do not offer freedom. Care is less about making good choices than rather about a concerted and ongoing process of calibrating and modulating existent technologies with present knowledge and its application to the complexity of diseased bodies. Drawing on ethnographic material collected in diabetes clinics in the Netherlands Mol argues, that good care is not necessarily enhanced by an increased or large variety of choices. Having more choices might not improve neither an individual's life, nor her or his care. Care has a logic of its own and what is understood as good care is dependent on local realities, local knowledge[5] and the given circumstances. While the two logics at times clash, Mol ascertains that they are also interdependent on one another (Mol 2008: 106).

In this chapter I aim to show that these two logics, the logic of care and the logic of choice, need a supplementation if we seek to grasp the dynamics that are at play before, during and after diagnoses of diabetes in a setting like Uganda. Here, access to diagnostics is not only a matter of care or choice. In settings like Uganda another logic is at play. A logic, which I will loosely come to term the logic of chance. I argue that a diagnosis is not only reliant on technology and knowledge in Uganda and it is not necessarily a matter of choice or money that buys quicker diagnoses and quicker access to diabetes care. Instead, whether or not a diagnosis is made possible, is also reliant on chances. The chance for instance to meet the right person in the right moment or the chance to access the right clinic with the right equipment and people that have the necessary knowledge.

In this chapter we will enter diagnostic spaces of different health facilities. The first two individuals we will meet, Judith and Mary, allow insights into two diagnostic journeys: Judith, who sought care in a governmental health facility and Mary in a private health facility. It will become apparent that the experiences before the time of a diagnosis are not that different between the two as would perhaps be expected. The last two sections will extend the diagnostic gaze and highlight aspects of diagnostic and testing practices in two governmental health facilities. We will see that chance is involved in diverse instances, which is then opened up for discussion in the last section of this chapter.

Diagnostic (un)certainties

I relished coming to health center IV in district Y nearly every Thursday morning. Not only was it one of the places I knew well, as I had already been here back in 2012 for previous studies. But it was the people who came here made these Thursday mornings so valuable. When in summer 2015 I came back for the first time, I was welcomed with joy, like a long-lost friend who had finally returned home. It never really felt like being at a hospital: trees were surrounding the small building, on about 60 square meters spread of land. Formerly a post for smallpox, it had been renovated ten years ago to accommodate this diabetes clinic. The atmosphere was relaxed. The individuals who came here for regular testing and checkup, too, seemed to enjoy the peacefulness of this calm place and the togetherness it provided. They lingered on the grass in front of the clinic after their appointments,

---

5   I follow Yanow's definition of local knowledge as "the very mundane, yet expert understanding of and practical reasoning about local conditions derived from lived experience" (Yanow 2004: 12).

chatting, laughing, exchanging and sharing their stories with each other. Though there were 418 patients registered, Sister Joy had organized the clinic days in such a way, that it rarely happened that patients waited longer than two hours before they were attended to. Stunningly little waiting time compared to other governmental health facilities I had visited. Often long waiting hours until an individual is attended to, sometimes a whole day, characterize most hospital visits. Surely this was also due to the fact that many health centers did not have a specialized diabetes clinic and patients had to wait next to individuals with other diseases, only to find out after hours of waiting that they had been waiting in vain: No technology for testing, no medication for treatment, and no prospect of improvement. The health center was a melting pot of people who had either already been diagnosed, those who were still waiting to be diagnosed and some individuals who left the clinic with the certainty of not having diabetes, at least for the time being. It was a governmental health center that was comparably well equipped with technology and a knowledgeable health worker.

Though I enjoyed coming to this hospital, it nevertheless still was a diabetes clinic. It was a facility where individuals came to seek help and care because they were suffering from an (un)known disease. A place, where many different stories and personal disease (hi)stories assembled; a place where the life of an individual could change with only one test. A life that, from the time a diagnosis of diabetes was pronounced, would mean a life with disease and a life in uncertainty. At the same time, it was a place, where some individuals finally found an answer to their pains after a long period of uncertainty. It is this clinic where I met Judith for the first time. The health center IV in district Y, however, was by no means the first clinic she had visited until she received her diagnosis. In fact, it did not only take her quite a long time to realize and perhaps avow herself that she might be ill. It also took a long time until she finally found out what was really wrong with her. One year of symptoms without diagnosis, visiting different health centers until she finally received a label, a name, a diagnosis.

Judith used to be a very strong lady. Since the death of her husband, she was the sole caregiver for her six children. Because the money she earned from selling the fruit and vegetables she was growing on her compound was not enough for a living, she took on additional work as a tailor. "Life was not easy after my husband died, but somehow we got around", she told me. Until in 2007 things started to change for the worse. Judith remembered: "In the beginning, I did not realize that I could be sick. You know, I did not expect a disease could be the reason for my thirst. But who would think that being thirsty too much is the sign of a disease?" The strong lady who she used to be, was soon replaced by a lady who felt weak. Her previously obese body turned slim and she started to fall sick time and again. A paralyzing weakness crawled into her body. Her thirst would not vanish. No matter how much water she drank it could simply not be quenched. At first the weakness came and went. There were still days, where she felt quite strong; but then the weakness stayed, sticking to every part of her enfeebled body. Every time she would sit down to take a rest, she felt her life fading away bit by bit. Feeling sick every day as soon as she woke up, she started to think that something was seriously wrong with her. Her first thought was that it must be malaria. It would not be the first time she suffered from malaria, "though if I think about it now, my body did not really feel like a body that had malaria. If I only had known that it was something bigger, I would have gone to the doctor earlier", she recalled. This is an aspect that a health worker once described to me too. Diabetes is a disease that often does not warn patients with painful or identifiable and rather known symptoms like fever. Instead, they live with the initial symptoms until the disease has already progressed. Diabetes often develops slowly, hidden, silent[6], and unrecognized. To say it in the words of Bury, chronic diseases "do not 'break-out' they 'creep up'" (Bury 1982: 170).

One morning, when she felt "extremely sick and close to death", she went to the next governmental health center to seek help there. One of her children had to accompany her because she was so weak she could barely walk alone. Supporting herself against the shoulder of her eldest son, she arrived at the hospital. After seeing a nurse in the outpatient ward, she was sent to the laboratory to be tested for malaria.[7] The test, however, turned out negative. Judith explained:

> "They simply sent me back home, because they said they would not know what else it could be. That was bad, because I had hoped for some medicine that could help me. That is why I thought if it would be malaria, it is nothing too bad, you can take medicine. You can cure it with medicine. I have had it before and know it well. I was desperate, because I felt something was really not right, but nobody could tell me what is going on. I had the feeling they were not taking me seriously. How could they just send me back home? I was obviously very sick and could hardly walk. Today, I think they sent me home because they simply did not know what to do with me and told me to leave because they were afraid I would just die on the spot in front of them and they wouldn't even know why".

The medical personnel at the health center told her to come back if the condition worsened, and it did. Only one week later, she found herself in the same outpatient department, waiting in the long queue for hours again to see a doctor or a nurse. Expecting to get an answer and hoping to get help. "This time they tested me for HIV. My husband had died from this disease and I had been tested several times

---

6 Since the symptoms of diabetes are often insidious, many people in Uganda have come to call diabetes "the silent killer".
7 The rapid diagnostic test (RDT) is one of the tests in Uganda, which is routinely performed to detect malaria; sometimes even then, when the symptoms are lacking that would hint at this disease. Though there are stock outs at times, it is frequently available even at lower health facilities.

before that, it has always been negative. But you can understand that I wanted to know? I wanted to understand what is wrong. I thought if it is HIV, then this is my fate. Then at least I would have known." When this test turned out negative, too, she was relieved and worried at the same time. Relieved, because she knew HIV was a "very bad disease", her husband had suffered unimaginably. Worried, because she still did not know what was wrong with her. "I was starting to doubt sanity. People did not believe me that I was sick, because I could not tell them what I was suffering from. Would you believe somebody being sick if she cannot tell you what the disease is called after a whole year of being sick and after being in different hospitals? Not knowing is not having it", she said shaking her head while remembering what had happened.

Subsequently, Judith went to two different governmental hospitals, receiving antibiotics and painkillers. But nothing helped and nobody could tell her what was plaguing her. It was not until she went to the fifth hospital, the health center IV in district Y, that she would finally hear a name for the disease that would change her life forever. Knowing the name of the disease that was causing all her pain: her weakness, her headaches, her excessive thirst and urination, her weight loss and her fears. Nevertheless, by the time her neighbors had rushed her to the health center, she was unconscious. Unconscious due to a diabetic shock: the levels of her blood glucose had dropped to life threatening values. "I was very lucky, that my neighbors found me and brought me here. I was already close to death. It was in this hospital where they tested me. That is when I was tested positive for diabetes."[8] Judith knew little about diabetes when her diagnosis was conveyed to her. Nobody in her family had it, as far as she knew. The only one she knew was her neighbor, the one who brought her to hospital. This, Judith was sure, had saved her life. "He knew the symptoms of a diabetic shock, he knew the disease and he knew where to take me. He acted fast and did not think long and brought me to this clinic where he himself had been diagnosed and where he is still treated." It is this health center, where Judith has come since.

Judith's story is no exception. I heard very similar narratives about the time before the diagnosis from other individuals. A time of false or simply absent diagnoses, treatment for allegedly present diseases and the long-lasting uncertainty what was really going on. One person I met for instance, a 54-year old man, visited nine different health centers over a period of two years. He was treated with antimalarial against malaria, antibiotics against a supposed bacterial infection and

---

8 "Testing positive" were words often used to refer to the diagnosis of diabetes. Positive or negative are terms, that are also used especially in HIV or malaria testing, where there are only two possible outcomes: either positive or negative (or of course invalid). Testing for diabetes, however, offers a range of different possibilities, as the outcome is not positive or negative, but it is a number.

with painkillers against his bodily aches. Like Judith, he was convinced that at times he would have been happier with an HIV diagnosis rather than continuing to live in uncertainty. By the time Joe was diagnosed with diabetes, his "eyes had turned black [blind]." A health worker stated that

> "even if you may think someone has diabetes you first need to investigate it with a diagnostic device in order to be able to confirm your diagnosis. The problem is, at many health facilities they do not even have the glucometer and in others they might have the glucometer, but you send somebody to the laboratory and the testing strips are not there. So how should we know it is really diabetes? We cannot diagnose whether or not a person has diabetes without it. People cannot simply base their diagnosis on signs and symptoms. Another very big problem is that the people are poor, so when they are told to go to private clinics for testing, they do not have the money. What they do then is simply go back home. What else should they do? It is a big problem and I can assure you it is not nice for us. Many treat diabetes as if it was malaria until they come here and we are investigating and find diabetes. But so many people are treated with antimalarial until we find out. It is a common practice".

A delay of timely diagnoses of diabetes can be related to a lack of knowledge about diabetes, respectively the correct interpretation of the insidious symptoms, especially at lower health facilities who are usually concerned with diseases such as malaria. When I visited a governmental health center III in a rural area of district X in my initial phase of research, the health worker in charge said "we health workers working in the governmental facilities are so stupid we have no idea about things. As long as I am not working on a disease, I will simply not know it. I am green [meaning she has no idea]. But who to blame? We know what we have been told and what we have in order to test." On the other hand, a diagnosis of diabetes is reliant on technology. Without a diagnostic device, it is simply not possible to uncover diabetes even if it is suspected. Judith knew that she was lucky that she had been diagnosed by chance. Not only lucky that she had finally found the answer to her pain and fears, but also the health center she attended was different from other health centers. This health center offered the feeling of community, she did not have to wait for long hours until it was her turn to see the diabetes nurse and she did not have to pay for treatment or the testing. She had access to the diabetes education classes taking place every second Friday of the month, where sister Joy educated them about the food they were allowed to eat, the food which they should avoid or eat in small portions. She had seen the importance of the glucometer in the process of receiving a diagnosis, because it was "the machine [glucometer] that had brought her diabetes". Though a life with diabetes was not easy, she felt taken care of, here at this health center.

We met Judith in this chapter. I have intended to show that individuals in Uganda often face long periods of diagnostic uncertainty when it comes to diagnosing diabetes in governmental facilities. Moreover, individuals may be confronted with false diagnoses and may be treated for diseases that are not the actual initiators for the symptoms, but are often based on presumptive diagnoses or what seems most probable and available. Judith went to five different governmental health facilities, received different medication – antimalarial, painkillers and antibiotics – before she was finally diagnosed with diabetes. If it hadn't been for her neighbor, who was able to recognize Judith's symptoms as diabetic symptoms and rushed her to a health facility, it could have turned out badly for her. It was by chance that factors came together that staved off the worst. We might now wonder, whether there is a difference between governmental and private health facilities in terms of access to diagnostics in the case of diabetes. Is the time of diagnostic uncertainty shortened when individuals are not reliant on governmental health facilities, because they have the financial means to access private facilities? These questions will be addressed in the following example where we will meet Mary who, unlike Judith, had money for a medical consultation at a private clinic and therefore supposedly easier and faster access to diagnostics.

Private Diagnostics

The national anthem of Uganda was resounding, the ringing tone of a mobile phone of one of the people waiting in the waiting area of this private diabetes clinic in Kampala. While I was waiting to meet one of the diabetes specialists and founder of the clinic, my eyes were roaming through the room. The small glass-topped tables positioned in front of the huge comfortable big black leather sofa lounge were still covered with a protective foil. Everything seemed to be brand-new here and indeed was. However, though it had opened its doors only recently, the number of diabetes patients registered at this private facility had already risen to 800. "Clients come here from all over the country, not only Ugandans but all nationalities. This is because the medical staff working here is specialized on diabetes", I was told by the receptionist. Information booklets from different glucometer production companies were neatly placed on top of the glass tables, ready to read them. Ready, to inform oneself about the newest technology available to monitor diabetes. A picture of Uganda's president, Yoweri Museveni, protected by a big, dark-wooded picture frame, was adorning the light-yellow painted wall of the waiting area. The stone floor was so brightly polished, that I was able to mirror myself in it – not a hint of dust, though it was dry season and dust usually found its way through the tiniest apertures. An air conditioner kept the heat out of the building. The receptionists were dressed in white polo shirts embroidered with the clinic-emblem, sitting behind the front desk right opposite of the entrance, welcoming some individuals, saying good bye to others, making appointments and cashing up the fees for consultation, examination and treatment.

Admittedly, this private clinic presented a very different picture from what I had seen before, even in other private clinics. The clinics own Facebook page included comments of people who had been to the clinic before or were frequently going there: "This is amazing, now this is the true steady progress. You and your loved ones don't have to fly abroad for these world class services, you can have the most qualified team of specialists in East Africa work on you right here in Kampala". Or "[g]reat services, lovely experience, caring people, with state of the art (high-Tech) medical machinery. This is what our country needs indeed", are two examples that reflected that I was not alone with my impression. With 50,000 UGX[9] only for consultation, 35,000 UGX[10] for an HbA1C test and 12,000 UGX[11] for a test with the glucometer[12], the prices, however, were rather high and beyond reach for many people. Compared to the health center IV in district Y, which had a diabetes clinic day only Thursdays, individuals were welcome to come on appointment or in acute situations daily between 9 a.m. and 7 p.m., except Sundays when the clinic was closed.

While this private facility had no problems with a lack of diagnostic devices and therefore diagnostic possibilities related to the uncovering of diabetes, it was not the first starting point of Mary's diagnostic journey, as we will come to see. Mary whom I met in this private clinic, too, described her story as one characterized by false diagnoses, mistaken treatments and the enduring and unbearable uncertainty of what was going on with her. There was, however, one difference between Judith from the first example and Mary: while Judith was reliant on governmental facilities where she would get free access to care, Mary had the means to go to private clinics for medical consultancy and care. She told me that she did not like governmental hospitals, where she would line up in the queue early in the morning only to leave it when the sun had started to set.

Diabetes was a disease that was not new to her. Her grandfather and an aunt from her mother's side both died from diabetes. Further, she had an uncle who was living with diabetes. However, as she told me, she did not mind about it too much before, because she never expected to have it herself. Mary explained:

---

9 Approximately 14 US Dollars.
10 Approximately 9,70 US Dollars, but the average price for this test even in governmental facilities if they offered this test, like the national referral hospital Mulago in Kampala.
11 Approximately 3,30 US Dollars.
12 Other private clinics I visited offered a test with the glucometer for 5,000 UGX (approximately 1,40 US Dollars).

"I never expected to have it myself, I didn't know, I didn't expect to get diabetes. I am a person who is scared and I let myself be tested as soon as I feel something is not right [...]. When it started [the diabetes] I didn't know that it was that. I had an itching in my private parts so I took all the other tests related to that. The doctors even gave me some medication against a vaginal yeast infection. Then there was a time where I was bleeding, I had heavy periods, very heavy and I didn't know what was wrong. I kept visiting the doctors and they would check and scan and check and scan, but they assured me that the results were always good. I didn't know it was diabetes that was disturbing me, but they [the doctors] didn't know either. After some time, I started experiencing more symptoms, my body would itch everywhere and when I came from taking a bath, my skin was so sensitive, I could not touch it without feeling a burn on that spot where I touched it. Sometimes I had to ask somebody to help me to scratch my back. It was itching everywhere, all the time. It was horrible. But each time I went to see the doctor, they would say that it is an allergy. The situation was getting bad, yet I wasn't getting to the bottom of the problem. This bleeding I was talking about, when I get the periods it is heavy. One week, second week, third week, I was given all these strong, strong medicines to stop it and gladly it did stop. But after some time, it turned out that even when it came to being with my husband [having sexual intercourse], then I would bleed. I would bleed, even when I was done with the periods and a week had passed or two. I think that is all from the diabetes, because they tell us wounds will not heal, so I think that was it. At the same time, I realized even in the sweetest fruit I used to enjoy, there wasn't the slightest sweetness. Even bananas. When it came to sweets, the taste was different, it had a funny taste. I said something must be the matter with my system, but I would go and complain to the doctors and each time they made all the tests and they did not reach a conclusion."

Mary was finally diagnosed with diabetes in a private clinic about one hour from Kampala close to where she lived. She told me that it was the glucometer with which the doctor found out that she had diabetes. When Mary's left foot started swelling and a wound on one of her toes was not healing, the infection spread quickly, and she could barely walk, she went to see the doctor. He pricked her swollen foot with a needle, but she was not feeling anything, her nerves were already damaged. It was hard to grasp for Mary that she should now have diabetes. She explained:

"It is not that I wasn't taking care of myself or I feared going to doctors or that I didn't have the money, I have it all. But still I got diabetes. I received education, what I have to do with the medicines and what I should eat. But what I didn't get is hope. I have the belief that it cures, that you can be free of diabetes. The doctor told me it is a chronic disease. You know what that means? So somehow, though I know better, I am still hoping for cure. For me it is not so easy, but since I don't want to get more problems I try my best."

As stated elsewhere, diabetes occurs everywhere, it can occur in any body and it is not bound to a specific geographic area or economic area nor is it necessarily connected to one's individual economy. It was her foot that brought her to this specialized diabetes clinic in Kampala. She was referred from her general doctor, because he said her foot had gotten so bad that he could not handle it any longer and specialists needed to take over. Now, being in this specialized clinic, it was not clear whether or not her damaged foot could be saved or if it would have to be amputated.[13] But Mary was convinced that this clinic could handle her disease in the best possible way, because here they had the best equipment, she told me. They did not only have glucometers but also "this big machine [HbA1C]"[14], which could show the glucose levels of the past three months, Mary explained. The pharmacy in the clinic was selling "the best available medicine for diabetes". But Mary had learned one thing about diabetes even before she was diagnosed "the best machines cannot help if diabetes is not found in time".

Mary, whom we have met in this section, does not distinguish herself much from Judith in terms of the time it took until she received a diagnosis. Both experienced a time of false diagnoses and mistaken treatments. The time before a diagnosis does not necessarily diverge much between individuals in Uganda, no matter how their economic standing is. The question posed initially of whether or not there might be a difference between governmental and private health facilities in terms of access to diagnostics in the case of diabetes can therefore for these examples clearly be answered with no. You do not necessarily have better access to diagnostics, respectively are able to avoid diagnostic detours in Uganda, if you have the financial means to visit private health facilities, where diagnostics are often perceived to be better. What differentiates the two, however, is the time *after* the diagnosis, where Mary had the chance to avoid tiresome waiting hours in governmental facilities and gain – or shall we say purchase – the feeling that the services she was accessing were the best possible. The following two sections, where we will enter two different governmental health facilities, intend to picture diagnostics from an additional perspective, namely the caregivers' side.

---

13 The diabetic foot is one side effect of uncontrolled diabetes. If the infection cannot be controlled and spreads, an amputation is often unavoidable.

14 The specialist working in this clinic told me that the HbA1C was the golden standard test they were using to diagnose diabetes. For a more detailed explanation of the different testing possibilities for diabetes, see chapter one.

Survival of the richest

It was a coincidence that brought me to the health center IV in district Z. Some friends had asked me to join them for an excursion to a village that was part of a sustainable building project. While they were busy with a tour through the village, I took the opportunity and visited the district's health center IV. It was located quite centrally on the margin of the district's main town. Only one week later I found myself in the diabetes clinic of this health center, where I met Sister Cathy, the head of the diabetes clinic. She told me that two years ago diabetes patients coming to the health center

> "were just handled by any clinician who was on duty. Most of the time somebody would just write down drugs and send a patient away. Some patients would even leave without knowing that they were having diabetes. Somebody would just come, say what the problem is and then be sent to the lab [laboratory]. If they found diabetes we would even write DM [diabetes] and inform the patient that you are a DM [diabetic]. But they were not told about food restrictions, about coming back for testing, no education at all. Somebody would go back and take the sugar. Somebody would go back and eat all the sugary things, taking sodas. They would continue eating their fatty oily things. When they came back again their condition had worsened. We actually diagnosed them again every time they came, because they simply did not understand what diabetes was, that it was chronic. Only telling someone he is diabetic is not enough. Diabetes is a very dangerous disease that has to be monitored regularly. Diabetes is a diagnosis that stays."

Care was formerly solely based on testing and providing medication, sometimes only medication (when the testing strips for the glucometer were unavailable). Individuals would go home after a diagnosis without knowing what this disease implied and what it meant to have a chronic disease, despite the fact the diabetes requires life-long medical attention. But things had changed. When I met Cathy for the first time, it had been exactly one year and eight months ago since the Medical Research Council (MRC) Uganda had come to the health center. They asked Cathy, if she could imagine being trained as a diabetes nurse in order to help initiate and then run a diabetes clinic as part of a pilot study. She did not hesitate to agree. She knew many individuals with diabetes. Not only here at the clinic, but also in her family and among her acquaintances. Around 124 individuals were registered in the diabetes clinic now, the number was increasing steadily. It was her duty as a nurse, she told me, to "save and serve", the slogan of nurses in Uganda. She knew that neglecting individuals affected with diabetes could be a death sentence for them.

I was not witnessing many diagnoses of diabetes myself, unlike HIV or malaria, where I saw people be labeled with these diseases almost daily. The reason for this is that most of the individuals I met throughout my studies in Uganda had already been diagnosed with diabetes prior to our first encounter. This made diagnosis appear as an a priori state, a seemingly uncontested and static given, which it of course was not. The few times I was present when an individual was diagnosed with diabetes, the testing procedure was rather unspectacular and quick: taking a tiny drop of blood, applying it to a glucose strip, inserting it into the glucometer and after only a few seconds the result – the blood sugar level – appeared on the screen in shape of a number. It seemed to be such a simple test compared to what it implied and entailed, namely a life with disease characterized by regular medical consultations and continuous testing. A diagnosis is one major break, but all the tests that follow can be seen as repeated caesura, especially when the result is undesired (meaning the number deviates from the normal values, either being too high or too low). As we will see throughout this book the chronicity and the longevity aspect of diabetes, makes the glucometer so essential in the handling of diabetes. The glucometer is the diagnostic device that on the one hand produced and produces individuals with diabetes, but on the other hand it often functioned as a co-creator of the stories we will come to read. It was what brought these narratives into being. It was what diagnosed the disease. Respectively, a diagnosis would not have been possible without it. It was, however, also the device, which was central for the continuous testing individuals with diabetes would be involved in.

The clinic took place every Monday from 8 a.m. (sometimes earlier, sometimes later) in a room close to the laboratory. This was useful, as the glucose levels of the individuals with diabetes would always have to be measured before patients would come for further consultation and for receiving medication from Cathy. Sometimes it was quite hard to climb over the legs of the people who were sitting along the narrow hallway. "The patients are too many", Cathy explained. There was hardly enough space to accommodate all of them in the hallway. Because the patients were so many, she would sometimes not finish her work until 6 p.m. Unlike Sister Joy whom we met before, Cathy was not only responsible for individuals affected with diabetes, but was working in different wards on different days: Mondays she was working in the diabetes clinic; Tuesdays, Wednesdays and Fridays she was busy in the general outpatient ward and Thursdays she was responsible for the ART clinic[15].

The handling of diabetes patients in terms of diagnosing and testing varied between the governmental health centers I had visited. While Sister Joy tested and treated her patients herself in only one room, other facilities collaborated with the laboratory and involved at least two different rooms and at least two people working on one person. Individuals would come to the health center and line up in front of

---

15 An ART clinic is a specialized clinic for the care and treatment of individuals affected by HIV.

the laboratory with other people who had come to be tested for all kinds of diseases. There they would be tested by a laboratory technician with a glucometer. After this, the glucose level in form of a number, would be noted in a patient book. The freshly tested individuals would carry the results to the health worker who took a look at the number, interpreted the blood glucose levels to finally decide how to proceed.

There were three different options: either a person was newly diagnosed with diabetes, or a person had already been diagnosed with diabetes previously and had come to the health facility for monitoring. Another possibility was that the glucose levels of an individual were unobtrusive, meaning no diabetes. In this health center IV, too, the testing ran in a different clinical space than the diabetes clinic, or rather the one room that functioned as the diabetes clinic. Testing was performed in the laboratory by a laboratory technician who used a glucometer. It was the glucometer the MRC had given Cathy. The MRC was also responsible for providing the testing strips and the pharmaceuticals. The consultation room was located at the end of the hallway, where Cathy would look at the numbers, speak out diagnoses or interpret testing results. She would prescribe and give out medication. It was her "every Monday business".

As mentioned, governmental health services are meant to be free in Uganda since the user fees had been abolished in 2001 (Meessen et al. 2006: 2253; see also the introduction). Since the MRC was providing all the supplies for the diabetes clinic – including glucose testing strips for the glucometer and all the required medicines – stock-outs rarely occurred. This was different from many governmental health facilities that were reliant on the supplies from the governmental body, the National Medical Stores (one example will be discussed shortly). At the health center IV in district Z all services in the diabetes clinic were free, too, attracting people to go there from other districts as well.

When I arrived at the health center one Monday morning, Cathy was not there as she was attending a workshop. On entering the room where the diabetes clinic was held, three people (one of them a medical student and the other two nursing students) were sitting behind the desk attending to a man. I knew the medical student from other times he had assisted Cathy because the workload had been too much. He told me right away that there were no strips for testing. Little did he know that Cathy usually kept the tin with the glucose strips in the desk drawer. In fact, Cathy told me later that she was hiding the vial of glucose testing strips because she did not trust the "lab guys" and did not want to leave it in the laboratory because she had heard that there was some "business made by selling the tests".

A patient confirmed Cathy's conjecture that the laboratory was making some business with glucose testing on the side. He said that when Cathy had not yet arrived in the mornings to take up her work, one of the guys from the laboratory would come to the people who were waiting to be tested and offered them to be tested right away if they paid 5,000 UGX[16]. 5,000 UGX and you could avoid standing in the long queue for many hours, sometimes the whole day. The patient clarified:

> "Before it used to be survival of the fittest. The ones who were strong could overtake the weaker ones in the queue so that they would leave the hospital earlier even than the ones who had already come very early in the morning. I did not like this behavior then, so I changed it by taking the lead and trying to control the queue and taking care that people would keep their spot and not overtake the weaker ones. But now it has become survival of the richest. The people who can pay the 5,000 UGX can simply overtake the people who do not have the money, and the lab guy [laboratory technician] even supports this, because he wants the money. The ones who pay the money, are the ones who go home early."

I did notice before that the laboratory technician had two glucometers on the table in the laboratory. But when I asked him why he had two, he simply told me that in case one of them broke he had another one he could use. I did not know at that point that one of the glucometers was his private one, which he used for testing his "clients" how he called the patients, who paid the 5,000 UGX. I would later observe a similar practice in other governmental health facilities too. A laboratory technician who was using the own glucometer in order to offer testing at the facility and with this circumventing the use of the facility-glucometer where testing was for free. Many patients were complaining that they were paying even when they did not decide to skip the queue. One laboratory technician who charged patients said: "Testing these people with diabetes is different than those other people. These DM's [diabetes patients] come back here regularly, I see them and test them regularly. I have the feeling they value the testing more and see the importance of testing if they pay for the test. Why not charge a small fee and get my share in this?" Later when I spoke to Cathy about it, she said:

> "You know, I did hear that in the lab [laboratory] there is some charging going on. That some people have to pay. All the services must be for free, but they charged them. But what shall I do? There is no other choice anyway. I told the lab that it is not correct what they are doing. But since we are not in the same room, I have no control over what they are doing. Only the patients can tell me later. It is in my mind that even if they charge, it is better than the patients going home not being tested. In private labs, the test sometimes even costs more than that, so they do save a bit of money compared to when I would send them away to be tested elsewhere."

---

16 Approximately 1,30 US Dollars.

On the one hand Cathy was glad that the labor was divided between the consultation of the patients and the testing. It meant a great relief against the backdrop of increasing numbers of people with diabetes attending the diabetes clinic, which she was in charge of by herself most of the times. On the other hand, it was exactly this division of labor, which made the charging by the laboratory technician possible in the first place. Cathy knew that the only way to bypass the extra-charging of her patients was to do both, perform the (diagnostic) testing as well as the consultations of her patients. "I will see that I get an expert patient so that he can help in the testing and then the people don't have to go to the lab. It will be better if I train somebody who can always help me in that field".

This third example brought us to the governmental health center IV in district Z. Compared to the health center IV in district Y, this facility had rather recently started offering services for individuals with diabetes, supported by the Medical Research Council of Uganda (compare chapter two). Unlike the first two empirical vignettes, where the diagnostic journeys of two individuals stood in the focus, this section intended to describe a facility where the access to the glucometer and therefore the possibility of testing and diagnosing diabetes was not only a matter of availability, but also a matter of in whose hands it was. We met a twofold logic of chance here: The chance of bypassing the long queue when paying a fee, but also the chance the laboratory technician took when charging the patients seeing the possibility to earn some extra money when Cathy, the in-charge of the diabetes clinic was not present. The last empirical example will bring us to a health center IV in district X, a governmental health facility where the diagnosis of diabetes has not been possible at all for the past months due to a lack of a glucometer and the matching testing strips and because of the wrong equipment ordering sheet.

Pending diagnoses and "technological flowers"

The health center IV in district X was located in the center of a town, a vibrant and busy place with big trucks passing through driving their goods to various destinations. The road passing by the health center was the main road connecting the West and the East of Uganda and therefore there was often traffic jam. I always enjoyed it much when it was the day to go there, mostly Tuesdays, though unlike the other two health centers, it did not have a specialized diabetes clinic or specialized health personnel. Perhaps this was also the reason, why nobody really knew how many individuals with diabetes were actually registered in the facility or who came for testing regularly. I remember when I came there one morning. A new consignment from the National Medical Stores (NMS) had reached the facility, like almost every second month. Huge boxes filled with sundry things that the hospital would need in the following time: pharmaceuticals, dressings, laboratory materials such as HIV testing kits, syphilis testing kits, cannula, rubber gloves etc. The storage manager of the hospital would manage the delivery and decide what was to be kept in stock in the hospital's storage room and what would be needed right away in the different wards, the laboratory or the pharmacy. He then distributed the commodities to the different wards. Eric, the head of the laboratory was awaiting the delivery desperately because he hoped to find two things in one of the big boxes: a new glucometer and the matching testing strips. It had been six months now that they had not been able to perform any glucose test, because NMS had failed to deliver a new glucometer and the matching strips. "This left many, many people undiagnosed, because even if diabetes is suspected, we still need to test. We sent some of the people to private laboratories in town to be tested from there, but many of them are poor and cannot afford the testing", Eric explained. His excitement while he was opening the boxes searching for these two things rubbed off on me. I stood beside him, my eyes trying to catch sight of something that could look like a glucometer or a box with glucose strips.

It was not the first time Eric had ordered a glucometer and testing strips. In fact, the laboratory had a glucometer, it even had five of them, but none of them was matching the testing strips that could be ordered on the ordering list from NMS. In one corner of the storage lying on the shelf board at eye height, there was a small collection of five glucometers of different brands. This was the glucometer graveyard of this health center. Glucometers that once fulfilled their duty, performing glucose tests, identifying individuals as having diabetes but that were now lying in the corner, non-functioning because the matching testing strips were missing. Eric himself could not recall where all of these glucometers had come from. Two came from NMS he was sure, but "the other three must have been donations or something. Glucometers come from abroad from people who have traveled or by foreigners who want to do good and help us with them. But it is a problem, because these brands they bring are not supported by NMS and therefore the testing strips are not available, and this is how we will collect the glucometers and keep them as technological flowers, because we cannot use them any longer." Eric, who was responsible for all the orders for the laboratory, told me that every time he had placed a new order for a glucometer and the matching strips, the next delivery came without these two things. He would be left disappointed again this time, there was neither a glucometer nor were there any testing strips in the box. He had checked the boxes thoroughly two times.

As hinted at, one of the problems why this health center IV in district X had so many glucometers was that they were reliant on which technologies would be supported and procured by the National Medical Stores. They had a standardized list of technologies, which would be distributed within Uganda to governmental health facilities.[17] In case of diabetes it was only one brand and type of glucometer, which was supported alongside the matching testing strips. I found out a bit later by an employee of NMS that the glucometer and the testing strips that were listed on the ordering sheet were no longer catered for. The company who used to produce the type of glucometer the health center was using had already developed "next generation glucometers". The model that was orderable was in fact obsolete. A problem, a mechanical engineer working for the Ministry of Health was well aware of:

> "Because of the global trends, it is the manufacturers of the glucometers who set the trends. It is not uncommon to find that many of the developing countries will end up with the highest standard technology for some diseases and with the lowest kind of technology of other diseases. The way these people are marketing technology now is that for them they come, pick a model and when they want to change it, they change it. Then they say, this is now obsolete we cannot support it, there are no spares. Like for the glucometer, they simply stop producing testing strips. They force you to move to the next generation technology. You will find that what is offered is always the state of the art. Even if you try to get the medium level, they will say 'no, in the next three years we are not going to support it. So we don't advise you to procure it.' Logically you will say, why should I get something which they are telling me I will get problems with getting spares. But then for instance the spare parts, the testing strips get even more expensive. For us what we need to learn is when you are procuring the equipment in itself is not the end of the discussion, we should look at the total lifecycle costs. You should look at what you need to have in order for the equipment to be used. The strips should be part of what you have to consider. Now, when you look at the procurement system that we are using for our medical supplies through NMS, there is a mismatch in terms of planning. NMS will say to our list of supplies, these are the strips we are going to have without taking a look at what is already there in the different health centers. Tomorrow you do procurement and you come with a totally different brand. It is a closed system, when NMS says they don't give you the strips or a new glucometer, they will not do it. 'Those ones, we even don't know about them, we cannot buy you the strips', something like that they would say. You might have a very nice glucometer, but you can't use it because you don't have any strips and NMS will refuse to buy. You will find very good equipment, but you can't use them because of a lack of small, small things."

The only thing Eric could respond to this after we chatted about NMS and the misleading ordering sheet was by asking "I am really wondering why they even

---

17 While NMS, the National Medical Stores are responsible for the governmental health facilities, JMS, the Joint Medical Stores procure and deliver to private health facilities.

put it on the list if it is no longer available? We are ordering and ordering and the glucometer we are so urgently in need of is not coming. Why?"

It is this fact, the interplay between the need to test people for diabetes, respectively to check their blood glucose levels, and the insecurity of whether or not a glucometer was and would be available and for how long it would remain useable, that fueled a certain phenomenon at this health center IV in district X (and elsewhere): the disappearance of glucometers. Eric told me that glucometers sometimes showed up at the hospital, "most likely donations from somewhere", only to disappear again shortly thereafter. Nobody knew where they had gone and who had taken them, though there were some assumptions. "It is mysterious. Like a glucometer atrophy", Eric said laughing. Yet his laughing could not overshadow that it also worried him. What should he tell all the people with diabetes who had come for testing? What about all those individuals in search and need for a diagnosis? Diabetes remains a disease where a diagnosis cannot merely be based on a presumptive diagnosis that may lead to a presumptive treatment.

I myself had brought a glucometer to the laboratory including 100 glucose testing strips, after the consignment from NMS came without it – that, however, was before I had learned about the vanishing of glucometers from the laboratory. I was all the more surprised, when the glucometer was gone a week later. When I asked one of the laboratory technicians where the glucometer was when I found it missing, she looked at me as if I was fooling her: "but you know we do not have a glucometer and we haven't tested any DM's [diabetes patients] for the past months". I told her about the glucometer I had brought to the health center the week before. "Who did you give it to?", she asked. When I told her that I didn't give it to a certain person, but to all the staff that was present that day, she replied "I am actually not wondering, some people come and take it and use it for their own lab [laboratory]. It is incredible, there are people suffering and still there are people from this hospital making money out of it. I was working from Monday to Sunday and I haven't seen the glucometer during this time." She told me that it was not uncommon that things disappeared from the laboratory. Many of the health workers, doctors or laboratory technicians were running private clinics next to their jobs at the governmental health center to supplement their low or pending salaries. "There is just no real control over the glucometer, especially if it is a donation. Then there is nothing much we can do", she explained.

This last empirical section brought us to a health center IV in district X and has pictured a facility struggling to deal with missing glucometers, matching testing strips, and therefore pending diagnoses. Like in the previous example we faced a double logic of chance. On the one hand diagnosis and testing was reliant on the chance that the ordering form listed the technologies (be it the strips or the glucometer itself) that match what is available in the laboratory. On the other hand, a laboratory technician took the chance making away with the glucometer to use it elsewhere. The following final section offers a platform to tie all the empirical examples together and to analyze how chance played a role in each one of them.

Diagnosis as a logic of chance?

Diagnosis is one of the first responses to suffering: the moment, when alleged certainty sets in and treatment can be brought on the way. It is the moment and practice that is universal across all diseases constituting the essence of most medical encounters. (Smith-Morris 2016: 1). As a diagnosis is the taxonomic tool of medicine it does what Bowker and Starr (1999) frame as 'work': "segmenting and ordering corporeal states, valorizing some, disregarding others, and in any case, exerting an important material force. A diagnosis is both the pre-existing set of categories agreed upon by the medical profession to designate a specific condition it considers pathological, and the process, or deliberate judgement, by which such a label is applied" (Bowker and Starr 1999, as cited in Jutel 2009: 278). It is the fundamental purpose of diagnosis to sort things out by identifying symptoms and ordering them into known disease categories (Smith-Morris 2016: 3). Labeling a person with a disease involves both, a process of sense-making of bodily symptoms, and a conclusion drawn thereafter.

As Helman (2007) points out, not every symptom an individual might experience can be translated into a diagnosis right away. Especially when a medical professional is not able to recognize and interpret bodily symptoms. Gill et al. (2009) relate severe complications of diabetes and its mortality rate of 10-30% in sub-Saharan Africa firstly to a delayed presentation to health care centers and secondly to misdiagnoses when patients are tested at the hospital (ibid.: 12). Burnam (1993) explains that "[m]ore often [as physicians,] we proximate meaning: rather than certitude, we deal with what is most likely. Inferring from the signs what might be wrong, we test for truth and discriminate among competing diagnostic possibilities by examining for the presence of a mosaic of harmonious signs that we might expect to find if our conjecture (or one of them) was tenable" (Burnam 1993: 941). Diagnoses, especially in severe and/or chronic conditions, is seldom made during the first visit to a health facility.

This chapter has pictured four different empirical vignettes, which were especially connected by one thing: diagnostics. As individuals suffering from (unexplainable) symptoms, we long for diagnostic certainty, we want to get rid of these symptoms and regain our health. The diagnosis of diabetes is not only a magical moment (in the sense that diagnostic certainty sets in) but also a shocking one: magical, because the moment initially holds a promise, the promise that there will be treatment and cure, especially after a long period of suffering without knowing the cause of ones' problems. Shocking especially then, when we may come to realize that the diagnosis we were longing for comes without these promises, without any hope for cure. As we have seen in the case of Mary, who, although she knew that diabetes is a chronic disease, still had hope to find a cure.

The possibility that symptoms are translated into a disease, which in the end proves wrong, has become apparent in the stories of Mary and Judith, who both experienced a long period of diagnostic uncertainty – a diagnostic odyssey with detours, characterized by a variety of false diagnoses. Though it was certainty the individuals sought, a name and a label, it was uncertainty that remained over an extended period. Even though Mary consulted different medical professionals in private facilities and Judith was reliant on governmental health services, both, Judith's as well as Mary's diagnostic journey stretched over a long period of time. Both sought consultation at different medical facilities until they finally gained the eagerly awaited diagnostic certainty. Judith stated that at times it would even have been better to be diagnosed with HIV, was not only a common statement I have heard also from other individuals with similar experiences, but shows how emotionally torturing diagnostic uncertainty can be. The third and fourth example finally, were told from a different stance, namely from the perspective of the care givers in two different governmental health facilities who are the ones in duty to provide the knowledge and the tools to test and diagnose diabetes. In the introduction of this chapter I have suggested that a diagnosis of diabetes is possible in the first place when knowledge and the necessary technologies come together in one place. If one of them is lacking, unavailable or unknown, a diagnosis remains both uncertain and nothing more than a (careful) approximation. However, even if technology and knowledge come together in one place, testing and diagnostic practices are not necessarily that straightforward in the case of diabetes.

As stated before Annemarie Mol (2008) contrasts two different ways of dealing with disease, which she has termed the logic of care and the logic of choice. The logic of care as the way we take care of our bodies in health and illness and that arises not from choices we make but from the practices in which we engage. In the logic of care, "care is an interactive, open-ended process that may be shaped and reshaped depending on its results" (ibid.: 20). The way a diseased body is taken care of is accordingly a matter of tuning, changing and adapting to the results that have evolved from care practices as a "try, adjust, try again" (ibid.). The logic of choice is contrastive to the logic of care and undermines patient care according to Mol. Especially in the minority world the neoliberal logic of choice is omnipresent in today's health care systems and has transformed individuals from patients into customers, who can "buy their care in exchange for money" (Mol 2008: 14). While the logic of choice leads us on that we have the freedom to choose what we think is best for us, it fails to acknowledge that in times of disease it is not all that easy to know what is really best for us, Mol argues. The wide array of choices – as good as they may seem in the beginning – can in fact be overwhelming. Being able to come to a decision can then be a complicated undertaking. Further, making a choice always involves that we are responsible for the consequences that can follow after we have made a choice, be it good or bad. Hereby, Mol specifies, choice "comes with many hierarchical dichotomies that are foreign to 'care': active versus passive; health versus disease; thinking versus action; will versus fate; mind versus body. Bringing these dichotomies into play is not going to improve the lives of people with a disease, if only because they end up time and again on the wrong side of the divide" (Mol 2008: 83f.).

Yet as João Biehl (2012) puts it, in "contexts of poverty, the financial and relational aspects of caregiving are often in extreme tension, placing people in very difficult situations in which they feel they have 'no choice'" (ibid.: 251). The logic of choice is not applicable in a setting like Uganda straightforwardly, where care is seriously curtailed by resource shortages, a lack of knowledges and a restricted way of being able to diagnose and later handle diabetes. My empirical material has complicated the neoliberal assumption that more money leads to more choices and therefore allegedly better care including a faster access to a diagnosis. Access to diagnostics and testing for diabetes, is not enhanced or even reliant on choices in Uganda. The empirical material instead suggests that it is always also a matter of chance whether or not an individual in Uganda will and can be diagnosed with diabetes, respectively if a caregiver can or is willing to diagnose or test her or his patients. A diagnosis of diabetes in Uganda, is not only reliant on the expertise of a medical professional and the availability of technology, but, as I argue, it is also a matter of chances; diagnosis follows the logic of chance. Which logics of chance then have become visible?

If we recall the first example, where we met Judith, it became clear that she, reliant on governmental health facilities that offered free care, had consulted different health facilities on different occasions. Neither of these facilities, for whatever reasons, was capable of diagnosing her with diabetes. Instead she was diagnosed and subsequently treated for other conditions until her health deteriorated to such an extent that she almost died. What saved her in the end was her knowledgeable neighbor. He himself suffered from diabetes and was alert when he found Judith and brought her to the right health facility that was able to test and treat her in the last minute – by chance. How about the second example, the story of Mary? Against the assumption of the logic of choice that an individual will be more independent, autonomous, and capable of acting, when there are different choices one can make, Mary also had a long period of diagnostic uncertainty and diagnostic detours. Though it was finally a private clinic where she received her diagnosis, other private clinics had previously failed to diagnose her. It seemed to make no difference whether she had the ability to pay for private services. Instead it is a common disease experience in diabetes everywhere, especially because the symptoms are insidious and sometimes tricky to identify as a symptom of an underlying disease.

It is an experience, which connects all individuals who are in search of a diagnosis – no matter whether they attend governmental or private health care facilities in Uganda or elsewhere.

Picturing these two stories of two women with a supposedly different financial background shows one thing quite clearly: being financially independent does not guarantee faster access to a diagnosis of diabetes in Uganda. It is not a matter of choice where to seek care. Rather it is the very chance of being in the right place, a facility able to provide appropriate diagnostic tools and the knowledge when and how to apply them; and the chance of meeting the right people at the right time. Meeting people, medical and non-medical individuals alike, who know how to recognize and interpret the symptoms of diabetes and therefore can initiate essential actions.

Yet what financial independency does influence is the time *after* a diagnosis of diabetes. While Mary and Judith had similar experiences in the time before the diagnosis in regard to the first symptoms and the diagnostic uncertainty, it was especially the time after the diagnosis, which differentiates the two and their disease experience: the feeling of what one thinks she or he can do about the disease when it is chronic in nature and therefore incurable. Mary had the means to handle her disease in what she considered the best possible way and consulted a specialist in one of the few specialized diabetes clinics in Uganda with the highest standard of technology available. Judith on the contrary was bound to governmental facilities, though the health center IV in district Y with its established diabetes clinic one day per week and experienced diabetes nurse, is clearly a place where knowledge and technology meet and interact effectively. What in this sense money can buy, is not the diagnosis itself, but for instance being able to avoid long waiting hours in overly crowded governmental health facilities. In the next chapter we will see that having the financial means further enables an individual to own a personal glucometer – like Mary who even owned two glucometers, or "machines" how Mary (and many others) called it. This is not only a way to monitor one's glucose levels, but is further a possibility to cope with chronic uncertainty that comes with diabetes and to regain a certain degree of control.

The last two examples hinted at a different aspect of diabetes testing and the standing and significance a glucometer has not only for the diagnosis of diabetes, but also (and perhaps even more so) for the time afterwards. Here the two examples occurred in two different governmental health facilities. In the first example, the laboratory technician was responsible for testing individuals who had come to the facility for being tested for and/or diagnosed with diabetes. The consultation and testing took place in two different places within the facility. This opened up the space and enhanced the chance for the laboratory technician who performed all glucose tests to translate the glucometer into a device, which would not only benefit the individuals who were tested, but also the laboratory technician himself. Without and against the permission of the in-charge of the diabetes clinic he charged a fee of 5,000 UGX for all individuals who wanted to, or rather could afford to be tested faster and skip the queue. At times it was, however, also possible that the laboratory technician charged any person whose glucose levels needed to be tested as soon as the in-charge was not present. That this was in fact not only against the will of the in-charge and the fellow patients, but against the governmental assurance that governmental health services should be offered for free, were subordinate for the laboratory technician. Presuming a price of 50,000 UGX[18] per can with 50 blood glucose testing strips (at times the price can even be up to 75,000 UGX[19] and more), this makes a profit of 120,000 UGX[20] per finished can. Against the backdrop of unpaid back wages, an attractive supplementary income.

Diabetes that comes with the need for long-term care changes the view a caregiver may have towards a patient. It was interesting that Cathy, but also sister Joy both spoke of patients, while, as soon as there was charging involved, the laboratory technicians both spoke of clients. The laboratory technician stated that not only the patients would benefit, but the laboratory technician profited too, a "win-win situation". Mol et al. postulate that "[f]raming care as a product for sale on a market makes it difficult to see that a lot of care work is not bought, but actually done by the patients. Far from just 'receiving' care, patients actively attend to their symptoms, swallow their pills, follow their diets, and so on [...]. Patients also actively visit their doctor – usually not because they freely 'choose' to shop for care, but rather because they 'have no option'" (Mol, Moser and Pols: 9). Because they have no option, as Mol et al. frames it, there is space for the care giver, a chance to transform the glucometer into a "money-making machine". It is a fact that patients with diabetes will have to be tested. There is simply no other alternative. In some of my empirical examples, the individuals changed from patient to consumer, but this happened involuntarily. In a market logic, the role of a consumer and costumer implies that a person has the choice to choose between an array of goods or services and exchanges money against either the good or the service. But in the case of governmental facilities the only possibilities to choose from in our third example was between paying the 5,000 UGX or going home untested and therefore either being left untreated or mistreated (when the medication cannot be adjusted due to missing glucose levels).

It is not my aim to pinpoint alleged professional misconduct in governmental health facilities, by either charging for tests that are meant to be free like in the third story or by purloining a glucometer in order to use it for one's own private clinic or oneself as in the fourth example. Instead I did want to hint at one very

---

18 Approximately 14 US Dollars.
19 Approximately 20 US Dollars.
20 Approximately 33 US Dollars.

specific aspect: the glucometer is a powerful device not only in relation to the uncovering of disease, but also in relation to how its purpose and use may be formed and altered to adapt to given circumstances and undefined as well as uncontrolled spaces. Since diabetes is a chronic disease, as soon as a diagnosis is established, and a treatment plan is brought on the way it is the beginning of a life in need of constant care without a choice of whether or not one wants to be tested. In acute, curable conditions, the interaction between patient and doctor usually ends as soon as the treatment has been successfully completed and an individual can be discharged symptomless and disease-free. However, since diabetes is a chronic disease, the diagnosis is merely the beginning. It forces into a life with disease that requires continuous testing. This has a great impact on an individual while at the same time opening up new spaces in relation to and in the handling of the glucometer. Testing, if you will, becomes chronic too, the glucometer functioning as the tool and motor. The glucometer draws its power from a reality of scarcity and limited availability, while it at the same time is the only means to uncover diabetes and to keep continuous testing going. When a diagnosis becomes a hard to obtain and retains desire (from individuals suffering from disease), the technology with which the diagnosis is taking place gains ever more meaning and opens up novel chances (for all actors involved who either use the technology or are reliant on it). It is then to a lesser extent a matter of choice than of chance that keeps care practices going.

As Mol and her colleagues aptly describe:

> Caring practices include technologies [...]. If they happen to be helpful, then they are welcome [...]. At the same time, engaging in care is not an innate human capacity or something everyone learns early on by imitating their mother. It is infused with experience and expertise and depends on subtle skills that may be adapted and improved along the way when they are attended to and when there is room for experimentation. Technologies, in their turn, are not as shiny, smooth and instrumental as they may be designed to look. Neither are they either straightforwardly effective on the one hand, or abject to failures on the other. Instead they tend to have a variety of effects. Some of these are predictable, while others are surprising. Technologies, what is more, do not work or fail in and of themselves. Rather, they depend on care work. On people willing to adapt their tools to a specific situation while adapting the situation to the tools, on and on, endlessly tinkering. (Mol, Moser and Pols 2010: 14f)

Instead of calling it a room for experimentation, in the case of the two governmental facilities I have presented, it was rather a room without control from the exterior, which made this experimentation possible. It then depends on what the caregivers or those in possession of the glucometer do with it, what they decide to use it for and especially where they decide to put it to use and under which conditions, rather than how and where it was meant to perform from the beginning. That an individual seeks a name for pain to finally be able to go on with life, and needs continuous testing to stay alive, hereby functions as a major driver for using the glucometer in profitable ways in governmental health centers, where exactly these tests with the glucometer should be free.

The logic of chance hovered next to the logic of care and the logic of choice in this chapter. Mol (2008) explicates that technologies are meant to create opportunities and not obligations. After the introduction of manufactured insulin, not injecting insulin for those dependent on it has become a lethal act and a therefore a moral activity at the same time. It is similar with the glucometer, though not using it is not a lethal act in itself, not having it, respectively not testing may lead to uncontrolled glucose levels, which in turn may be lethal. It is this fact that has created a space for using the glucometer differently. For the care-seeker it is the choice between being tested for 5,000 UGX or not testing at all, but also a matter of finances and therefore of chance. For the care-giver it is the chance of receiving 5,000 UGX per test or not, but he or she is left unharmed even if an individual decides not to pay. But it is often not the individuals themselves who have the choice whether or not to be tested, and it is not only the care givers who have it in their hands, but there are bigger forces at play. It is an entanglement of structural, social, individual and technological circumstances that may promote and facilitate or prevent practices.

The last example was taken from a health center IV in district X, a health facility where no glucose tests could be performed during the past six months. NMS, the responsible governmental body for the procurement and distribution of medical technologies in Uganda, neither provided a new glucometer nor glucose testing strips that matched the device that was already there. The mismatching of technology (outdated technology listed on the ordering sheet though it in fact it is no longer produced) or the glucometer graveyards that buried different devices that would still function if the matching strips were available, added up to the complexity of diagnosing and testing for diabetes in governmental facilities. The chance here lay in having the right ordering sheet, or by chance having a donated glucometer which was matching the strips that were orderable.

In chapter two, I have illustrated that diabetes is as a disease, which is still in the making in Uganda (and elsewhere). Lacking policies and guidelines on the one hand and a slowly adapting health care system in terms of providing the necessary tools (glucometers and glucose strips, guidelines and policies) on the other hand, made it possible that there is an uncontrolled influx of technology, of which nobody knew where it came from or by whom. Whoever abstracted the glucometer from the laboratory – though it is hard to speak of stealing as the device was nobodies designated property – saw a chance of taking the device and applying it to another place without being charged for it or even recognized by others. It was a donation, a gift, and neither the property of the health facility nor of a specific person per se. As this technology is undocumented in the official recording system of the health center, it is easy to take away donated technology unnoticed. Donated technology or private technology brought to a governmental facility is beyond the control of any government or hospital authority. Who would miss the glucometer and who was to blame if it was gone? Who would have the authority to restrict testing practices with the private devices of a laboratory technician charging for his 'work' if he or she was filling a testing and diagnostic gap for the case of diabetes because the Ministry of Health was not providing it? Though the glucometer had been "abducted" it most likely was continuing to do its care-work elsewhere – either for self-monitoring practices or in a private clinic, perhaps in a village where the next facility with a glucometer was far away.

Diabetes fosters unpredictable and unknown practices that at times bring glucometers to health facilities or at times take them away from there. It is this technology-shortage, which increases the desire to possess it. Where care generally is reliant on the availability of technologies and choice is limited to what is provided, a logic of chance, I suggest, links both. It grapples diabetes, its diagnosis and the continuous testing as a chance to keep the glucometer and therefore testing, diagnostics and care going. In short: a diagnosis of diabetes in Uganda is clearly a matter of technology and knowledge coming together in one place. But a diagnosis and the testing of this disease always also follows a logic of chance: meeting the right people at the right time; being in the right place; having the right ordering sheet or glucose testing strips that match the glucometer. Nevertheless, diagnosis is also dependent on in whose hands the glucometer lies in and what this person decides to do with it and which chances to take or to omit.

6. My numbers and my-Self

What is a number, really? In this chapter, I aim to showcase the power of numbers. The world we are living in today is, perhaps as never before, a world in which quantifications and metrics take on an imperative role. We live in a "world of numbers" (Diaz-Bone and Didier 2016), in a "world of indicators" (Rottenburg et al. 2015), and in a world, in which what counts in global and public health is "metrics" (Adams 2016). Accordingly, we may express ourselves or may be expressed through numbers. A number measures something or rather is a symbol and result of measuring something. It represents an amount and/or a quantity; it gives a picture of something and it clearly most often stands for something. I think we agree that no matter for what we may use a number, it will not have a deeper meaning unless you, or someone adds this meaning to it. Numbers have to be related to something or some-body, and whoever uses them has to have an understanding or the authority to interpret and analyze this number in order to make it useful in one way or the other. A number might be an abstract or empty entity for one person, while it may mean the world for another.

Numbers have the power to influence important decisions, thoughts and even our feelings. They are seen to be a way to block out the (often unwanted) subjectivity of narratives and stories and are taken to be matter of facts, stable and certain entities (Neyland 2013: 220), such as in evidence-based medicine (chapter three). Though numbers lead us on to be neutral, they by no means are, as we have seen and will come to see. Numbers have a value and not only the value ascribed to a digit in terms of quantity, but "[t]he way in which phenomena are quantified and interpreted and the purposes to which these measurements are put are always implicated in social relationships, power dynamics and ways of seeing" (Lupton 2016: 96; cf. Nielsen and Grøn 2013: 56f.). How may we give meaning and come to understand parts of who we are and how we feel through numbers? In the case of diabetes, the number emerging from self-monitoring practices with the help of a glucometer, functions as representation of the bodily state in which an individual finds her- or himself, which cannot be visualized and identified or made knowable in quantitative terms otherwise. Nielsen and Grøn (2013) state, referring to Hacking (2002)

> [n]umbers indicate if something is more or less, but also better or worse than something else. Therefore, the number not only represents a numerical value, but also a normative value. The number is bestowed [in] the ability to reflect who we are, in what direction we are heading and how well we behave [...]. [N]umbers are not neutral and solely meaningful within a biomedical treatment regimen, but [...] numbers" [and with this the glucometers as transporters and producers of these numbers] "can become normative devices in patients' pursuit of happiness, health, and the good life. (ibid.: 62f.)

Thus far I have spoken of numbers and metrics and the knowledge and authority that may be drawn from them in order to inform policies and bring medical interventions on the way in the realm of global and public health. In this chapter I intend to zoom in and shed light on what numbers, or a very certain number for that matter, might mean for an individual. For numbers do not only have a collective significance, but also an individual one. The glucometer hereby is not only a producer of knowledge about populations the way Umlauf (2017) argued, but also functions as a device to produce knowledge about one's self. To be precise: which meaning, emotions or translations and what knowledge may an individual in Uganda who engages in self-monitoring practices ascribe to and gain from certain numbers emerging from (self-) testing? How may a number be translated into lived reality? That is, those few who own a glucometer and put it to use to measure their glucose levels and with this seek to control 'their' diabetes. But also, how may the understanding of one and the same number diverge in its use and interpretation between medical professionals and their patients?

The numbers we will come to meet in this chapter are not the numbers used to monitor or surveil a group of people (previous chapter). Instead we will look at numbers and the meaning ascribed to them for the life and the self-monitoring practices of the "everyday life worlds of ordinary people" (Diaz-Bone and Didier 2016: 6). The glucometer hereby is not only a means to quantify glucose by displaying a number on a display, but also a mediator and negotiator of and to control diabetes: it entails a paradox of being controlled through the glucometer while simultaneously seeking to gain control through the glucometer that shall be pictured throughout the following narratives. I argue that while indeed it is the number that counts in self-monitoring practices, it cannot be separated from the medium, the glucometer, with which it is produced. The glucometer has a dual character as it is a device holding the power to limit uncertainty (by making the glucose levels and therefore the bodily condition visible) and to gain control over a disease in a body that is out-of-control. At the same time, it is the object and source of uncertainty ("When will I be able to test myself again?"). The glucometer does not work on its own, but individuals will need resources in order to put it to work – in a setting with weak infrastructures and a limited availability of resources often a difficult undertaking.

It is assumed that self-monitoring will bring more awareness and certainty about the disease when translating subjectivity – a symptom or bodily sensation – into supposed objectivity, by utilizing the glucometer in order to make this subjective sensation measurable, quantifiable and visible through a number. The glucometer attempts to "penetrate the dark interior of the body and to render it visible, knowable and thereby (it is assumed) manageable" (Lupton 2016: 54; chapter five). The number hereby may provide essential information concerning the correlation between diet, physical activity and the intake of medication with (too) high or (too) low blood sugar levels. Nevertheless, it is also seen to be fundamental for preventing harmful outcomes of continuously uncontrolled glucose levels, which may lead to medical complications (e.g. kidney failure, loss of sight, amputations etc.) or even death (chapter one). On the other hand, next to assessing the success of the treatment regimen, a medical person may also utilize the numbers deriving from testing to limit the time spent on each individual for the glucometer does exactly that, translates subjective conduct into a seemingly objectively quantified number.

For individuals relying on insulin for survival, or for those with a great variation of glucose levels, self-monitoring is not only essential, but indispensable. The (scientific) dispute over whether self-monitoring has the same positive and significant effects in individuals with type 2 diabetes, respectively those who do not utilize insulin but are on oral medication, is ongoing (cf. Klonoff 2008; Farmer et al. 2009).[1] In other words: in the world of global health and its reliance on evidence and metrics, significant evidence is lacking that proves self-monitoring of blood glucose to be a truly beneficial practice for an individual to engage in.[2] For individuals on oral medication the usefulness of self-monitoring has been questioned. Generally, it is only useful "when results are reviewed and acted upon by healthcare providers and/or people with diabetes to actively modify behaviour and/or adjust treatment" (IDF 2009: 4; see also IDF 2008). Nevertheless, it *can* be a useful supplement for successful disease management (Kirk and Stegner 2010: 435). I propose and aim to show in this chapter, that self-monitoring can be especially beneficial in settings with weak health infrastructures. Settings, where testing is not only a

---

1 Most of the studies conducted on self-monitoring of individuals with type 2 diabetes are located in the minority world, where health infrastructures are stable and in case of an emergency medical attention and care can be sought rather quickly.
2 In Germany, the lacking evidence of the usefulness of self-monitoring in individuals with type 2 diabetes is a reason for health insurances not to cover the costs arising from these practices, for instance when purchasing testing strips for patients. There are, however, voices underlining the comforting and beneficial effect of self-monitoring as an essential tool, which should be made available to all patients independent from their diabetes type and medication status (cf. Czupryniak et al. 2014).

matter of usefulness or willingness, but a matter of access to and availability of resources required for testing. In Uganda, it is often not possible to be tested more than once in a month or even every second month. Or, as it was often the case, not at all due to a stock-out of testing strips or missing glucometers at a governmental health facility (chapter five). The number arising from (self-)testing here is, unlike in settings where frequent measurements are possible even several times a day, the fulcrum around which care has to be organized for a long period of time.

Following Lupton (2016), as she is referring to the influential and much-debated work of Foucault on selfhood and technologies of the self (1986/1988)[3], in different eras, different ideas, discourses and expectations circulate in a society. How individuals ought to behave and should conduct themselves, is hereby internalized through practices geared towards the care of the self (Lupton 2016: 46). Technologies of the self is a notion, which ascribes more agency to an individual instead of staging her or him as a person utterly dependent on the state. Empowered individuals choose and immerse themselves in practices in pursuit of their own interests and desires, as a person capable of deciding what is best for her or him (Lupton 2016: 48; Guell 2009). Surely, self-monitoring and caring for the self in a cooperation between individual and caregiver has become an essential tool in the new global health where chronic diseases are located in the realm of care and not of cure (Guell 2012; Lupton 1995). Lupton states that in

> contemporary western societies, the care of the self is viewed as an ethical project, which requires self-awareness based on critical and considered reflection and the acquisition of self-knowledge as part of achieving the ideal of the 'good citizen' – that is, a citizen who is responsible, capable and self-regulated in the pursuit of happiness, health, productivity and well-being [...] [P]eople must take responsibility for the outcomes of their lives. (Lupton 2016: 46f.)

The expectation and the practices involved to satisfy these expectations are extended and no longer merely lie in the hands of medical professionals. But patients suffering from a chronic disease are equally expected to take good care of themselves and do everything it takes to maintain a stable health condition. In the case of diabetes this may include changing nutritional habits, engaging in exercise or,

---

3 With his earlier concept of bio-power Foucault names one function of the modern state as the "administration of bodies and the calculated management of life" (Foucault 1979: 139f.) staging the human body as "a site of power enactments and struggles" (Lupton 2016: 52). Bio-power hereby includes how human beings attend to their bodies and the ways in which they manage and regulate them, as well as how they are monitored and the wellbeing of a population may be promoted and achieved. "Rather than disciplinary power being exerted on individuals or populations, biopower is exerted, not only by government authorities but by the range of other agencies that focus on humans' bodies and behaviours, such as commercial and research enterprises" (ibid.).

as will be the center of the following empirical vignettes from Uganda, self-monitor one's blood glucose if possible.[4] Though the notion of technologies of the self seems applicable to this book, I intend to view self-monitoring practices of individuals not as "ethical exercise" or an "ethical project" maintaining good health and therefore being a "good citizen". Instead, and in line with Guell (2009; 2012), I will view self-monitoring as a practice to diminish uncertainty and regain hope and safety for the future and keep death at a distance (Guell 2009: 3).

The advances in medical technology gain a new implication especially in the case of chronic disease.

> Part of this increasing use of visualising technologies is a significant shift in how the body and health states are conceptualised, articulated, and portrayed. Where once people relied upon the sensations they felt in their bodies and reported to their physicians, medical technologies devoted to producing images of the body have altered the experience and treatment of bodies. (Lupton 2016: 53)

Here it is not only the medical practitioner who uses the glucometer in a clinical setting in order to measure one's glucose levels and let them guide the treatment and medical trajectories and procedures. It is the patients themselves who are (and must be) active to complement the collection of numbers – from their homes or wherever they decide to measure. A locational shift from the laboratory or a medicalized space, to an individual's home; a shift in responsibilities from the professional to the lay person; and a shift in the temporal dimension, from measuring only when coming to a health facility, to measuring whenever it seems necessary. However, self-monitoring entails expectations, which many individuals in Uganda cannot live up to, respectively individuals will have to find their ways to include self-monitoring in their lives in ways that suit their needs and preconditions.

As we have already seen in chapter four, the introduction of glucometers has not only come with new possibilities of dealing with disease. The self-use of these technologies has brought along new obligations. The obligation, now having to take care of oneself without the assistance of a medical professional, alongside the requirement to produce valuable and correct results, which can later be made productive. At the same time individuals have to be able to understand these numbers, interpret them correctly and translate them into appropriate action: do more sports,

---

4 As mentioned elsewhere exercise and changes in diet can have a great impact on the glucose levels of an individual who has diabetes. The reason why I am not focusing on these measures to self-care is simply due to the fact that firstly exercising was not common among the individuals I met. Further, changes in diet (here I am not speaking of omitting sugar, which most of the individuals do as soon as they hear they have diabetes) are not a simple task. In settings where there is a scarcity of foods any way and the variety of what to eat is limited, to change the nutrition is, as I was told by many of my informants, often impossible. "What do they expect me to do, eat the leaves of the tree?", as one of the individuals I once met ironically asked.

increase the dose of medication, adjust the diet when the glucose levels are high, take some sugar in cases of low blood sugar, etc. As Mol described it for the case of the Netherlands:

> [T]he self must come to behave like a professional. This begins in self-monitoring, where one must become one's own laboratory technician and adopt the necessary skills: to be accurate when measuring, to use the right amount of blood, to properly write down the numbers. For some people that's being professional enough [...]. Thus, with this small diagnostic device, the miniature blood sugar measurement machine [glucometer] that allows one to measure the blood sugar level of one's own body, patients gain independence from professionals. But they do so at the price of taking over professional skills and tasks. (Mol 2000: 18f.)

In Uganda, individuals who engage in self-testing do take on professional tasks. But producing numbers outside the clinical setting is also a way of substituting the lack of resources in governmental facilities. Diabetes offers an interesting case for the use of medical technology, as a glucometer assists in the production and gathering of data about oneself, or a certain group of people (individuals with diabetes). It further "orients the medical action taken on a specific patient and acts as the basis for aggregate-level investigations, and for new therapies and diagnostic procedures. The reliability, truthfulness, and accuracy of such information is therefore of crucial importance for healthcare practitioners. Accordingly, being able to count on 'empowered' patients is the best way to obtain reliable, detailed, and updated data" (Bruni and Rizzi 2013: 29). The movement from being a patient who relies on the care and testing of and through medical personnel to becoming a patient who actively takes care of one's self, may alter the way in which an individual comes to understand a disease and in consequence parts of the self. The ontology of the glucometer, alongside the numbers it produces, can illuminate ways of dealing with and doing disease – a perspective that has largely gone unquestioned for under resourced settings until now.

The success of diabetes self-care is highly reliant on subjective infrastructures: Individuals will need the knowledge and the resources to what it takes to perform and interpret the results of self-testing, act upon them and have the constant access to technologies that enable these practices and keep them going. In the case of diabetes self-monitoring in Uganda, care practices are not only a practice of measuring glucose levels and acting upon the results. Individuals bargain and tinker while their lives are fundamentally molded by the disease and what they think they can do with what they have to control it (Guell 2009: 21). This chapter aims at displaying narratives of people who are in one way or the other involved in self-monitoring. We will read when and how they (can) use the glucometer, what the device means to them and how the number determines their life worlds, feelings and thoughts. In the first empirical part of this chapter I will describe how a caregiver perceives the usefulness and meaning of self-monitoring of her patients for her own work.

"Numbers don't lie"

It was a beautiful early morning on this Thursday when I arrived at the health center at around 7 o'clock – like almost every Thursday. That was the day the diabetes clinic was held, which I knew quite well by now, since I had already spent a lot of time there during my very first stay in Uganda. It was a well attuned practice: I would arrive at the health center, park the car underneath a tree, and then walk up a narrow short and stony mud path passing the main hospital building on the right-hand side until I would reach three small houses standing about five meters away from each other. Some of the hospital staff was living there, the lucky ones, sparing them from tiresome trips to this small town located about 30 minutes away from Kampala. Like Sister Joy, the head nurse of the diabetes clinic, whom I was going to pick up. Joy was heading the diabetes clinic already since 2007, and was an expert in field, having attended several trainings on diabetes care and diabetes management in Uganda and abroad. Her house was the one in the middle, the one with the purple curtains and a floral print. I would knock at the door and Sister Joy would welcome me with a cup of milk tea, which we would drink while sitting on the steps in front of house. A good start to the day and a few minutes' time to chat before we would then walk the short distance to the small diabetes clinic, a three-minute walk from there. Sister Joy was carrying a big red plastic bag filled with the new consignment that had been delivered this week: boxes with medication. When we approached the clinic on this Thursday morning, two ladies were already waiting in front of the clinic waving and smiling at us. Sister Joy took out a set of keys and opened the big padlock of the metal door. It was the same procedure every Thursday: opening the clinic, entering, pulling back the white curtains in the waiting room and the examination room[5], the walls embellished with posters picturing diabetes related topics in Luganda (the diabetic foot, where to inject insulin or the food guide pyramid). Then preparing everything for this clinic day. This involved getting all the things for the examination of the patients from the big wooden cabinet and placing them neatly and ready to use on the wooden desk: boxes of medicine, the blood pressure machine, the tin with the testing strips, the documentation books "Improving Health Services Response to Chronic Diseases" and of course the glucometer. The device, which "made us capture many patients

---

[5] The small building comprised only these two rooms, the anteroom, where the patients would sit on wooden benches waiting for their turn and the examination room.

who did not know they had diabetes", Joy commented while stacking the meanwhile nine documentation books filled with names and numbers. The glucometer was "a hard-working machine", which made Joy's work a lot easier as she was able to assess how patients were "really doing". When Joy sat down behind desk ready for the clinic day to begin, she told me that "[t]hings were going bad for the people lately, many of the patients were having bad glucose readings with very high numbers." She understood this as the outcome of the fears of death the individuals were having, especially when one of their fellow patients had passed away. "They now fear the same will happen to them", she said.

The diabetes clinic, which was actually a combination of a diabetes and hypertension clinic[6], always started early in the mornings around 7.30 o'clock. The patients with diabetes were requested to come for the testing before they had breakfast, because "food has an impact on the glucose levels". Joy did not want her patients to wait too long to prevent their glucose levels from dropping too much. One by one the waiting room of the clinic was filling up. When the first patient, a young lady, came into the consultation room she took a seat on the chair next to Joy's desk and handed over diabetes association member card. Most of the patients attending her clinic were part of the clinic's own diabetes association, which Joy brought into being some years ago. Patients who were members or wanted to become members of this association had to pay a yearly fee of 30.000 UGX[7] and in turn were provided with medication and received glucose testing in times of supply shortages of the government. Additionally, they received a membership card in which the appointments were noted as well as the testing results.

"I tell the patients to carry the membership card with them everywhere they go. In case of emergency, when they fall into a coma or are unable to talk, people will find the card and are able to identify them as DMs [diabetics]. This way the doctors can act fast and also see the last glucose readings in case they might not have a glucometer to test them", she explained. Joy took the membership card of the lady and unfolded it. Joy's eyes got big: "Why did you not come to your appointment on the 17th of July? When we give you an appointment, make sure you come, understand?", Joy asked with an angry undertone. Joy always got very angry, or rather she seemed angry but was actually rather worried. "Some of these people simply do not take diabetes serious enough. If they don't come to their appointments like I tell them, this means they sometimes are not monitored for three months. This

---

6 Diabetes and hypertension are seen as two diseases "moving together", meaning that individuals who have diabetes often also have hypertension and vice versa. Therefore, it is common practice to combine the clinics for these two conditions to ease the handling (monitoring and management of the diseases) for both, the patient and the health professional.
7 Approximately 8,20 US Dollars.

is way too long, especially for those who do not have the glucometer at home and that is the majority of the DMs."

Having to take care of around 418 diabetes patients[8] in total and sometimes more than 35 patients on a clinic day, required a bit of strictness she explained. Otherwise the patients would end up dying one after the other – that was her experience after being trained as a diabetes nurse more than ten years ago. She had seen many patients during this time, some of them died and some of them were in a bad medical condition, because they were not able to monitor themselves at home, and then some of them were not even showing up for the appointments. "Now, what do you expect me to do? It means I am just joking with somebody's life if I do not take my work seriously and try to make the situation clear for my patients." After working with diabetes patients for such a long time, Sister Joy felt disillusioned sometimes. She saw patients suffering, but hands were tied if they did not help in order for to be able to help them. She explicated:

> "You know, self-monitoring with a glucometer at home is an important aspect of the care of a diabetes patient here in Uganda. You see, some patients come here every other month, which means they will only be tested six times in a whole year. This again means I only have six wimpy numbers that tell me how much medicine to prescribe, and how a patient is really doing medical wise. This is not enough. Now imagine, the ones who can afford self-monitoring, even the ones who might only test once every two weeks, they will have four times as many numbers in one year. But these numbers are the only thing that helps me to control my patients. It is not the things they tell me, no, it is the numbers. Anything that happens in the time without testing, you must consider yourself not being safe, if you do not test. You simply do not know what is happening with yourself. But when you have your glucometer and you feel unwell, you would know now I am in this level and let me manage according to the teachings I get. If everyone would do self-monitoring, I am sure there would be no problem, but testing on a monthly or even two months' basis is simply not enough."

Every time an individual entered the examination room, sitting down, handing over the membership card where the results and the next appointment would be noted down, willingly holding out one finger to be pricked, Sister Joy would ask: "You tell me the range in which the result should now be in?" Nearly every individual would give the same answer: "Between four and seven"[9]. Each time these words would be said, words which were hovering through the examination room like a

---

8 I counted them personally by going through the nine documentation books. However, there is the likelihood that some of the registered people dropped out or died in the course of time.
9 The complete designation including the unit of measurement would include millimoles per liter [mmol/L] stated after the number.

holy mantra, Sister Joy would nod approvingly and then turn over the glucometer so that the individual was able to read the result on the screen. If a patient could not give an answer, she said the numbers a couple of times – "between four and seven, between four and seven..." and then let the individual repeat the words. Was the result in the range, Sister Joy was obviously relieved, but if it was not, she said "Now look at this. This is not a good number, look closely, can you see it? It means you are not well controlled, you are in danger and your life is in danger, do you understand?".

The numbers, Joy explained, were an indicator and a window through which she could "look into the inner body" of an individual and the glucometer was "assistant". She needed the number to know patients. "Numbers don't lie, but sometimes patients do", she insinuated. Sometimes she would ask an individual before she started testing how she was doing. According to Joy some of patients would exaggerate, trying to tell that they felt very bad and that they had the feeling they were in a bad state. The test result, however, proved otherwise. The opposite was possible too, that a person would claim to feel great, not having any symptoms or feeling sick, but the number reflected a different situation. It was important for Joy to be able to draw a correlation between how each of patients was feeling, or claimed they would be feeling, and the result, the number that then appeared on the glucometer. For if the feeling deviated too much from the test result, she knew that in times where she was not able to test due to a lack of testing strips, she would not rely too much on what an individual was saying: "You know, I have to get to know my patients. Each of them is different, has a different personality, and each of them handles the disease in a different way. I have to be able to know them, if they are weaker or stronger in what they can endure. If I cannot test them, I will be more careful in changing the doses of the medication. If I am in doubt, I will rather leave the medication as it was."

She was sure that it was a big advantage if an individual was able to afford to self-monitor. She was then not forced to rely on gut instincts in case the glucometer was out of function, but could draw on the numbers the individuals had documented at home. Patients would not get into the danger zone of hypoglycemia (too low blood sugar) or hyperglycemia (too high blood sugar) so quickly for they were able to act upon the numbers even though she was not around. Especially hypoglycemia would kill fast if not counteracted. Patients were educated about the dangers of too high and too low blood sugars and the symptoms they could expect for either state. Having to rely on the correct interpretation of the bodily symptoms of either too high or too low glucose levels was tricky and at times dangerous. If a person would think she was in a state of too low blood sugar and then eat or drink something sweet to bring the levels back up, while actually in a state of too high blood sugar, this could cost a life or induce irreducible damages to the body:

"If someone does self-monitoring I can better control this patient because I am helped to control this person".

Nevertheless, Joy knew that only very few of patients actually owned a glucometer, let alone that they were able to monitor themselves regularly or even several times a day. In fact, only around 11 patients out of the 418 patients self-monitored regularly[10], Joy told me. Regularly was a wide term, "it is also regular in a way, when a patient tests once every month", she commented. Most of them were unable to afford the high costs of maintaining this practice. Yet compared to the city with a rather high density of private and governmental medical facilities it was the people living in remote areas, where the next health center was often far away, who could profit immensely and where a "glucometer could really save a life, it is a life-saver". Measuring the glucose level only once a month could not be a substitute for the time between the appointments. It meant the loss of many numbers, numbers that would have helped and patients to understand the current state and the development of the disease. One month could be a really long time, a long time in which the glucose levels could go beyond the range.

Though Sister Joy trusted the results of the glucometer, she trusted the one she was using at the diabetes clinic more, or rather it was the way she was using it, she trusted more, she told me. It is not only the object (glucometer) that is important. The knowledge when and how to use the tool, as well as the willingness to stay as objective as possible, even if the numbers displayed by the glucometer are not pleasant to read for the patient, are equally important. Some of the patients who were self-monitoring were not using the glucometer correctly, not storing the strips properly, and not "following the simple guidelines and therefore producing incorrect numbers". Others, she was thinking, might simply make up a number, write down "a fake number" to please and not make angry. In fact, I had a conversation with a patient once, who confirmed Sister Joy's assumption stating that "if I have too bad numbers I sometimes write something else in my book because I know Sister will get angry with me." Sometimes she had patients who showed their little booklet in which they wrote their results they had collected at home. While the numbers in the booklet only showed numbers that were in the range, they were "hyper, hyper, hyper", meaning having an overly high glucose level when she tested them at the diabetes clinic, which made wonder whether they performed the tests correctly, the device was faulty, or they were making up numbers. She had to retest patients, when she did not trust the results they were bringing. "If you see the diary

---

10 The ideal case in Joy's eyes was to test three times a day: one time before breakfast, then before lunch or alternatively before dinner and then before going to bed – on a daily basis. Testing six times a day, 42 times a week and 168 times a month would mean an enormous financial burden. One test costing around 3.000 UGX, makes 504.000 UGX every month, which is around 131 US Dollars per month and 1572 US Dollars in one year.

some of the patients keep and you doubt the numbers then you retest and use your own glucometer, because you know that yours is well kept and is in good condition and of course that you have no reason to fake a number. I do not always trust the people. It is a tough situation, because I should trust my patients and create trust. But my years as a nurse have shown that numbers don't lie, but the people who are expected to bring me these numbers do sometimes, I am sure."

It was now 11 o'clock and the 28 patients who had attended the clinic that day had all gone. Joy and I were still in the examination room clearing up. The small boxes of medicine, the non-communicable diseases registration books, the glucometer and the last tin left with glucose strips had to be put back into the big wooden cabinet standing next to the window, which would be locked afterwards – all things waiting to be taken out again the next Thursday for the next diabetes clinic. Empty medicine boxes were thrown into the garbage. While we were tidying, Joy and I were chatting sorting numerous boxes of the new medicine from the red plastic bag she had carried in the morning into the drawers and shelves of the big wooden cabinet standing in the corner of the examination room. To make things easier I grabbed some of the boxes and handed them over to Joy who then neatly placed them into the cabinet. When the bag was empty, Joy asked with astonishment: "Are there no strips?" The bag was empty. Joy went to desk, took the small tin with glucose strips and shook it tenderly to hear how many strips could be left. There were not many strips left, certainly not enough for the next diabetes clinic. "See, that is the reality. Sometimes I can test and then there are times where I cannot. That's how it is. As much as I like my assistant the glucometer, it is only useful as long as the strips are there and as long as it can make me some numbers."

In this section we have met Sister Joy, the head nurse of the diabetes clinic. Though she encourages her patients to self-monitor as a way to help her do her work, we have also seen that she at times mistrusts her patients and the results they bring. Like Joy said, the numbers were a way to know how her patients were really doing healthwise, but also a way to get to know the personality of her patients and assess whether they were trustworthy or not. That self-monitoring can have a beneficial effect on the self-confidence and self-understanding of individuals who have fallen ill with diabetes will become apparent in the following two sections.

Knowing the good number

The laboratory technician of health center B was excited when he came up to me while I was sitting on the bench in the laboratory taking some notes, sitting next to people who were waiting to be tested for all kinds of different diseases. "Oh, Arlena, look there, this is one of our DMs [diabetics] back there. His name is Josh", he said. There was indeed reason to be excited, especially for me, Josh was exceptional. There were not many patients with diabetes registered at Health Center B, compared to the other places I frequently visited – possibly a result from an absent specialized diabetes clinic at his health center. After the laboratory technician introduced us to each other we started chatting, while the usual laboratory business was going on in the background. The glucometer was hidden in a little green plastic basket on the laboratory bench, covered by rapid diagnostic tests for malaria, HIV quick-tests, paper and other things. But Josh apparently knew where to find the glucometer. I was watching him, while he started testing himself. This was a rather unusual sight for me that he tested *himself* instead of being tested by one of the laboratory technicians like the other patients. He told me that he always came to this health center and preferred testing himself, given that the strips were there. Since he came every other day, everybody knew him well and there was no need for him to wait in the queue. Versed in doing so, he ripped open the paper of a blood lancet, pricked himself in the side of his middle finger[11], filled the testing strip with the tiny droplet of blood and waited a few seconds until he heard the glucometer beep. Then he checked which number the glucometer indicated on the small screen and imparted the result to the laboratory technician who wrote the number into the big outpatient registration book: 8.1 mmol/L. Next to his name, his village, his age and his sex. 8.1 mmol/L was what the glucometer had displayed. "What does that number mean?", I asked Josh. "Well, this is a very good number and it means I am doing just fine."[12]

Having been in touch all along, I was finally to meet Josh one year after our first encounter at health center B. I visited Josh at his home where I also met his wife with whom he had been married for many years and with whom he has a little daughter. Josh seemed to be a very busy man: pastor of his own church, a businessman owning a catering service and having initiated a circle for microfinance, called the *Living Gospel Circle*. Josh turned 34 in 2017 and he told me that he enjoys reading books, any kind of book or magazine. But what he loves reading most is anything he has searched on the Internet, because "Google is [his] friend". Because he loves to read, it came to him naturally to search the Internet when he started experiencing "weird" symptoms and changes in his body. That was in 2014. Perhaps unlike many others to whom the diagnosis of diabetes comes as a shock and surprise, Josh had expected it. He expected that one day he would have diabetes. Diabetes was the disease both of his parents had died from. He told me that he remembered very vividly that he was praying when he started typing the two words

---

[11] It is recommended not to prick into the fingertip, but the side of the finger instead due to sensational problems that might occur after some time, as the nerves get damaged during the course of the disease.
[12] According to the American Diabetes Association a glucose level of 8.1 mmol/L is already elevated.

diabetes and *symptoms* into the Google search engine. He prayed that the symptoms that would be displayed on the screen after he pressed the enter key would not match the symptoms he was currently experiencing. His fears, however, were to become reality: the symptoms of diabetes described on the screen did match.

Josh recalled that everything started with his sight. He woke up one day with a blurred vision. "I got worried because I remember my mom kept saying, she was getting a blurred vision." Having parents who both suffered from diabetes he had "a constant fear in [his] heart of getting diabetes". He explained "I think this is one of the reasons why I got it this early. You know when you are always in a worry, in stress and working hard, you have a family at a tender age [...]. I was going through a lot in a short time." He went to Health Center B, the closest governmental health center, to seek consultation and to find a clear answer to his question "Was I really having diabetes?". When he came to the health center, the medical officer who attended to him sent him to the laboratory for further investigations.

> "The doctor was shocked when he saw the testing results and requested me to go back for a fasting blood sugar test[13] the next day and I remember it was 14.4 [mmol/L]. I did not sleep that night; I was worried and was thinking, 'ok, I am finished'. I was always in fear, in that constant fear of getting this disease. So anytime I got sick, and even if it could have been something completely different, I first thought it was diabetes. As soon as my little finger was itching, I thought of diabetes. My head was simply locked there. But still it is something else to have this fear in your head than when it becomes real."

Everything Josh knew, he had learned from the Internet or from what he still remembered from his parents. It was also in the Internet where he read about the importance of monitoring the blood sugar levels daily. Even though the time we first met, Josh went to Health Center B to monitor his glucose levels, he got fed up after some time because it had been too many times that he went there, only to find that the strips were out of stock. Moreover, the staff was "too busy performing malaria tests" or not having the necessary expertise to deal with diabetes.

> "You know, the attitude is terrible, they do not have eyes for people with diabetes like me. Some just don't know what diabetes is. Then there are people who check you and they are putting a certain look on their faces, which could kill you. They are just not qualified. Sometimes I went to these private laboratories and was just teaching those people what to do and what the numbers mean. Someone is checking you, and they see it [the sugar level] is 6 and they say 'a little high'. You start wondering if what you know is true [...]. Finally, you discover that they do

---

13 A fasting blood sugar test refers to testing the blood sugar in a body state in which the person has not eaten for at least 8 hours; otherwise the blood sugar level would be referred to as random (see also chapter one).

not even know what they are talking about. 6 [mmol/L] is a good number and they should really know this. Even if it is 9 [mmol/L] it is ok, if they check you randomly."

He decided to stop going there. Since he could spare some money, he decided to start self-monitoring at home instead, exactly like he had read on the Internet. In contrast to most of the other individuals with diabetes, Josh was not taking any medication to keep his sugar levels stable. He explained that when he took the medication, he experienced a lot of hypoglycemia (too low blood sugar). Instead of using tablets, he regulated his sugar levels only with exercise and diet.[14] This at least was the case most of the time. The exception was that he started using tablets again when going through stressful times as his "numbers would not go back to normal without it". Or when he had very high glucose levels and feared he could not control it otherwise. In those phases, he measured very diligently.

Josh usually tested himself three times a day. Sometimes even four times or more. But "always in the morning", he said, for "that one is a must". When he had many testing strips, however, he constantly checked himself and carried his machine everywhere. He did not care how people reacted when he tested himself in a matatu[15] or somewhere else in public. It was an emergency situation he wanted to prevent. "I am the kind of person who checks myself whenever I do not feel well, maybe I feel shaky or something, so I do not want to waste too much time thinking about the reasons. When you are shaking, you do not know if the blood sugar is high or low, because for me it is the same sign. It is tricky and it is confusing. It is only through testing and the number I get that I will really know what is going on. It is the only way to know if I have a good number or a bad number and how bad it really is." It has happened once that Josh ran out of strips, unable to pursue his daily routine of testing several times. Since he was not testing and was unable to know his glucose levels, he started drinking soda when he thought his glucose levels were low, though in fact they were high: "I did not know what is happening, because the signs are the same, that is the tricky bit of diabetes, the signs are sometimes the same when it is low and when it is high, so you do not know, you cannot tell really." Now whenever he ran out of strips and he could not afford to buy them out of his own pocket, he immediately went to his friends and asked them for money, or borrowed money from the circle, the micro-finance association he had initiated. As soon as he had some extra money to spare, he tried to stock the strips, to avoid running into the same situation.

Josh was lucky. He did not have to pay for the glucometer he was using. A laboratory technician gave it to him in a private laboratory. They had a promotion

---

14 In fact, Josh was the only person I met during my research, who was not using any medication at all and the only one regulating his sugar levels merely with diet and physical activities.
15 A matatu is a minibus and one of the main public transport vehicles in Uganda.

where only the strips had to be bought while the glucometer was given out for free[16], "that is how lucky I got, maybe for people to find out that this is a good glucometer, they were marketing themselves", Josh reasoned. He was very satisfied with his glucometer, he thought it was a good brand. Since he had some contacts, he could buy 50 testing strips for 50.000 UGX[17]. "That's a good price", Josh said, knowing that there were many people who could not afford paying this price and "that this was what was killing people, because they just cannot afford."

It is health status[18], the glucometer gave, Josh said, and it was what he needed "to know myself". He rather checked his glucose level with the machine than merely listening to his body symptoms, though listening to his body would perhaps propel him to test even more, he speculated. He loved his glucometer, because it generated numbers and these numbers were a guidance, a pointer in which direction to go and what to do and this made his life easier. The number encouraged him to do more exercise when it was high and it gave him the "permission" to rest and take it easy when it was low. If he went through periods of "hypo"[19], he could even allow himself to take some soda or eat a few fatty things. It had another great asset: when the number was in the range, it told him what he himself could never know without it and that made him happy.

But having a glucometer, Josh knew, had both, positive as well as negative effects. It was not the testing itself Josh really feared. As long as the numbers on the display were good, he felt good, but when it was not good, he got scared and for this he sometimes feared the numbers: Moments of frustration, when the glucometer showed a high result for example. There was a time in which he was experiencing periods of high sugar levels no matter when he would test. He got fed up and did not want to use the glucometer any longer. "Even if you had all the money in the world", he said, you will not be "able to buy good numbers". He wanted to throw the glucometer away or hide it so that he would not have to look at it. Not testing was a way of not having to know, not having to deal with at times unwanted and frightening numbers. Until he realized that it was himself who was able to control his life with the glucometer, exercising more, living a healthier lifestyle without drinking too much alcohol or eating fatty foods or sweets. He was able to control his numbers, and not letting the numbers control him. The glucometer could only

---

16 As we have seen earlier, this is common practice in much of the minority world today that pharmaceutical companies give out free meters.
17 Approximately 13,70 US Dollars.
18 Though for some patients it is exactly status, which the glucometer brings. Not only health status, but status in the sense that only individuals with money are able to afford to buy and maintain a glucometer.
19 "Hypo" is the abbreviation often used by people with diabetes or medical professionals referring to hypoglycemia, too low blood sugar levels. "Hyper" on the contrary relates to hyperglycemia, too high blood sugar levels.

assist him, but it could not take the work out of his hands, which would have to follow after the testing. What the glucometer helped him with was to know what to do and what not to do. It also helped him to assess if what he was feeling was right or wrong or close to the testing result or far off. Though having a glucometer made him think about diabetes a lot, he was certain that he thought about diabetes in a good way, because "you use the glucometer and this glucometer brings a number and this number makes you think about your life. You know, diabetes is a condition which is supposed to be thought about. You should think about it and monitor it, that means you should watch it. Do not allow the numbers to stress you, but think about them. The glucometer always reminds me, if I should ever forget to take good care of myself."

During one of our interviews, when Josh grabbed his backpack, which was placed next to his desk in the small office of the church, opened it and pulled out his glucometer. It was neatly stored inside a small black nylon case, prevented from falling out with a black rubber strap. Then he tested himself: 8.5 mmol/L. "A very good number", Josh said. Josh knew quite well which numbers were good and which ones worrying, something he shared with his fellow patients. Knowing the good numbers was something most individuals with diabetes were very aware of, though the range could differ. This is why Josh had his very own good number. It was good to have one number, a "magic number", that served as the goal one could strive for. A good number that, when achieved, should make one proud and happy. For Josh this good number was the number 8. "I am not sure if it is really a good number for other people who have diabetes too. But for me it is the number when I feel great. This number brings me comfort and calms me down if I am in fear of death. If I am desperate and fearful, even if it is nothing to do with diabetes, and I test and I have an 8, my fears vanish behind this number."

Next to measuring the glucose levels for mere medical reasons, Josh mentioned another feature the numbers brought along with them: "I think there is a psychological attachment to the number on the meter." When the glucometer displays a good number, he felt happy. When it was high, he would get worried:

> "When you see good numbers day in day out, you might even get a diabetes burnout, that is you start forgetting that you are supposed to live a certain lifestyle. Then you go back to eating meat and chicken and sugar and you take a little wine […]. Others just get tired of it and they say, 'ah, that is too much pricking every time'. I have a friend of mine called Moses, he gets the machine and throws it away and says 'I am not going to be a slave of diabetes'. For me it is not about being a slave, but simply the wish not to die from diabetes early."

Without the glucometer it was hard to know whether the levels were high or low. But with the glucometer, one would easily be able to identify the levels and know how to act accordingly, without having to go to the hospital. "Diabetes is a permanent damage of life. You cannot do things the way others do them. I read a lot about how a patient can live with diabetes because now I am part of it, I cannot escape from it. If people would want to 'act normal' without testing, they might die, since they cannot see with their eyes how the sugar is moving in their blood. But the glucometer performs magic. You cannot look into your body, but with the glucometer you can."

Josh was certain that it was the knowledge people in Uganda were lacking. The knowledge about what individuals with diabetes could do to make their lives easier. "My bible says the people perish because of lack of knowledge. Knowledge is very important, so what is going to help people with diabetes in Uganda is knowledge. People should know. One part of this knowledge is the knowledge about yourself. It might one day save their life." That is why he would never stop testing, "because testing my blood sugar is one way of knowing myself", Josh said.

Josh in this section used the glucometer in order to test himself as a means to circumvent to be reliant on the health care at governmental facilities with which he was not satisfied. The glucometer was a way to be in control over his situation himself avoiding tiresome visits to hospitals where the medical staff seemed to be unknowledgeable. Having a glucometer further provided him with a good feeling when the number was good, and he was able to counteract bad glucose readings. Such as taking something sugary to bring the glucose levels back up. The next empirical vignette will introduce Elizabeth to you, who, like Josh, owned a glucometer and engaged in self-monitoring. For her owning a glucometer is a way of living a better life, because it becomes more predictable through testing the glucose levels regularly.

"Who shall I trust more, the number or myself?"

Turning left into a small path branching off from the main road, we, my research assistant and I, drove about ten minutes along a narrow and bumpy path, the tires of the car blowing up the dust from the ground, which had not seen rain in days. It was the usual practice that when we had an appointment for an interview at an individual's home, we had to call the interviewee on our way to get directions. It was not always easy to maneuver through villages without street names or distinct landmarks for orientation – though we often lost our way, we also always found it in the end. While I was driving, my interpreter was on the phone translating the directions: "Turn left where they are selling the tomatoes" or "now we have to slope left and pass the avocado tree", she directed me. When we arrived, Elizabeth was already waiting for us by the roadside, waving while still holding her mobile phone in her left hand. I met Elizabeth for the first time in the summer of 2015 at the diabetes clinic of the health center IV in district Y. I still remember the day very well, when I came to the clinic, seeing Elizabeth joyfully together with two other women, fanning herself with a sheet of creased checked paper to make the air move that seemed to stand still. Elizabeth lived in a small house together with her husband and her two children in a populous neighborhood. She kept poultry and did some farming, growing pineapples, bananas and some maize for a living. Most of the pineapples and bananas would be sold on the market and after harvesting the maize would be dried in the sun to be taken to a milling machine later on, which made maize flour out of it. She had prepared a nice shady spot in front of her house and welcomed us to have a seat on one of the white plastic chairs she had nicely arranged beforehand. Chickens were running around in the yard chased by a rooster; children's laughter was echoing in the distance.

Elizabeth told me that she was not the only one in her family who had diabetes. Her brother who followed her as the eighth child, too, had been suffering from it, but died in hospital. It was now ten years ago, since she started experiencing first symptoms: frequent urination and excessive thirst. She became tired very fast and always felt weak. When she went to a health center to find out what was plaguing her, the nurse told her she would be tested for four diseases: Brucella, typhoid, HIV and diabetes. Elizabeth did not know why exactly those four diseases, but after she had been tested for the first three diseases, all results turned out negative. Subsequently she was sent to the diabetes clinic of the health center IV in district Y for the last test. "If this test turns out negative" she remembered the nurse telling her "then I have no other idea what you are suffering from". The nurse at the diabetes clinic, Sister Joy, whom we have met in the first empirical vignette of this chapter, started asking questions such as: "Do you see very well?" Elizabeth replied that she saw well. "Are you the one who brought yourself here?" Elizabeth answered that yes, she came by herself. Sister Joy explained Elizabeth that she had never seen before what she saw on that very day – the glucometer failed to give numbers as the glucose level seemed to be too high for the machine to be able to measure it[20]. That day Elizabeth was admitted to hospital and this was also the day after which Elizabeth would not be able to live the life she had lived before, it was the day "when my life would be determined by the fear of death and numbers".

Like Josh, Elizabeth too was "one of these lucky people" who had a glucometer at home with which she could engage in self-monitoring. She tested between two and four times a day, depending on her situation. The meter was given to her for free at the diabetes clinic, because she was a good friend to one of the nurses who

---

20 A glucometer can only display glucose levels for a certain range. If the level of glucose exceeds this range in either extreme high or extreme low levels, it usually indicates "HI" for high or an Error for both, too high and too low levels. Depending on the brand and type of glucometer the cutoff usually lies between 28 mmol/L and 33 mmol/L for the high levels – a life-threatening glucose level, which requires immediate medical attention and action (see also chapter five).

was involved in the diabetes project for children, the ones with type 1 diabetes. Since she had "a good connection to the nurse" the strips were given out for free too, at least most of the time when she needed more.[21]

> "You know, I consider myself to be a lucky person, because I received the [gluco]meter for free. Usually these health workers assume that type 2 patients are adults, grown-up people who are expected to be working and can afford to buy meters for themselves. The hospital is making charity to the children who cannot afford buying meters for themselves to ease their life. When you are young they think you are a bit irresponsible, so they will have to think for you sometimes, but for the adults the moment you know that you need something, you are somehow expected to make sure that you get it, because the moment you don't take it [diabetes] serious you start thinking of what life for your family will be after your death, how should the people you have been looking after sustain themselves if you don't take care of yourself?"

Before Elizabeth got the glucometer, she always had to "guess the number". She could get symptoms like feeling heavy, her bones aching, or feeling dizzy. Then she started guessing what the number could be if she would measure her glucose level at that point. At times it was hard for her to know whether the way she was feeling was the result of a too high or too low glucose level or whether it was something different that was bothering her. "If I was in worries over something that happened in my life, if a friend died or I had a fight with one of my children, I could feel it in my body. I did not know if it was the diabetes or other worries that people have once in a while too. There are people who are afraid and their heart beats fast, and they do not have diabetes." Then there were times, in which the number displayed on the glucometer at the health center did not at all match the way she was feeling. The nurse always told her, that she should trust her feeling because she was not able to measure her glucose levels. But "who should I trust more", Elizabeth asked me "my number or myself?" When the number deviated too much from the feeling she had in her body, she thought, then it must be the feeling that is wrong and not the number. But then again, if her feeling was not wrong, but the number, then was it not possible "that I do not have diabetes but something else. But would the doctor use the glucometer if it makes wrong numbers?" The time without a glucometer was a very confusing time for Elizabeth. It was hard for her to trust herself and her feelings in the face of often conflicting numbers. She remembered that she used to admire the people who had a glucometer at home. They could always check and

---

21 Novo Nordisk, a Danish pharmaceutical company has initiated a project "Changing diabetes in children", which provided free meters, testing strips an insulin to children and adolescents with type 1 diabetes. For more information on this initiative, see: https://www.novonordisk.com/sustainability/actions/Access-to-care/CDiC.html.

verify their feelings. She instead had to speculate and guess, live in uncertainty and confusion. "If you do not know your number all the time when you feel confusion or if you have symptoms, everything you will be doing is a risk and a danger. You might just eat whatever you want. You will start getting these wrong thoughts, which I had, when I was wondering if I even have the disease or not."

The situation changed when Elizabeth received her glucometer. She realized that the more she tested herself, the more the numbers on the display of the glucometer started to match the way she was feeling. It was in a way that Elizabeth learned a lot about herself, when it was a feeling that was related to diabetes and when it was not. She was for instance able to see the immediate effect of her insulin injections on the number. She saw that when she ate and injected herself according to the readings on the glucometer, she was not only rewarded with stable glucose levels, a fact that had gone unseen, even confused her, until then. But she also felt "peace" because she was able to know her status at any time, especially in moments where she was unable to differentiate the symptoms as effects of too high or too low blood sugar levels, as we have also seen in the case of Josh. When Elizabeth woke up one morning, shortly after she had received the glucometer, she felt free knowing "I had the meter to know my numbers whenever I feel bad". The glucometer gave her hope to "live a better life", a life beyond moments of uncertainty such as fluctuating glucose levels and the confusing unpredictability of how the disease may develop, but also how to interpret bodily symptoms. As Elizabeth put it

> "diabetes changes like weather, which can be complicated; like now the sun is shining, within one minute it may change to being cloudy or even rain. It is the same with diabetes, you might test in the morning or even after eating and find out that the number is good, but by the time you go to sleep you are badly off and are close to dying. [...] Regular testing helps me to keep away or at least recognize instabilities."

The beauty about the machine, Elizabeth said, was also that it would not need a lot of time to perform the test, all the same it would not require a lot of knowledge to use it. Elizabeth felt like she had become a "doctor to [her]self", which gave her confidence on the one hand but also the freedom to travel to the village again where parts of her family lived, where hospitals or doctors were often far away. It helped her to "monitor life" and assisted her in knowing what was going on within her body. Especially when it would come to emergency situations, the glucometer would be of help: "If you have the machine you will be monitoring your life [...]. Patients who do not have the machine will have to predict their blood sugar statuses like I did before. With the machine [glucometer] you stop estimating and predicting, you will know your status, because you see it through the number."

Though Elizabeth always carried along the glucometer, she usually only tested from home: in the morning when she woke up, to "know her number that starts her day", then either before or after lunch, sometimes before supper, and the last testing was done before she went to bed. The doctor would see her as careless and irresponsible with her life if she did not test. She had the machine and therefore no excuse for why she could not test like others did. Testing was important especially before she went to bed, because many people would die at night during their sleep.[22] That is why Elizabeth felt worried and stressed sometimes, when the glucometer displayed a high number. But then she was able to inject a dose of insulin to make it drop again and therefore the glucometer gave her some sense of being in charge and control over her own life. It also offered her the prospect of "living a better life" – if a life with diabetes, then a more predictable one. In order to prevent death, she had to test regularly whereby "the glucometer gives me hope and safety for life because with it I will know how my life stands […], this will make me increase on the chances of staying alive, if I do not have the machine I will not know, there will be no way I can monitor my life and this will put me in much danger. That is why they say poor people die in a worse state compared to the rich because if you can afford buying the machine and monitor your life, you cannot have a mysterious death."

Elizabeth described how much better it was to engage in self-testing than merely rely on the testing in a hospital:

> "I felt better than when I go to the doctor. Most times patients fear to go the doctors because doctors sometimes get rude to the patients more so when they find that your numbers are bad. They take you to be reluctant and careless with your life, so to make you maintain the status, they have to be rude. This makes patients become afraid of going to the hospitals, but if you have your machine and you test from your home, you will be free from such frustrations. When your number is high you will know, and find ways of reducing it before going to the doctor. Also, when you know your number and can tell the doctor this number, you will not have to use many words and spend too much time on describing the way you feel, but the number says more than all my words would be able to say. Even among my friend with diabetes I can simply tell them my number and they will know if I feel good or bad."

She saw it as her responsibility to be able to know her status, while the doctor was professionally accountable for (medical) situations she could not handle. Continuous testing was her duty but also a privilege as compared to patients without meter, as at any moment their condition could worsen without them knowing.

---

22 What Elizabeth is referring to is known as the so-called 'dead-in-bed-syndrome' and describes the death of a young individual with type 1 diabetes who did not have a history of long-term complications, respectively did not show any signs or symptoms for complications before going to bed (O'Reilly et al. 2010: 585).

There was another responsibility Elizabeth described. Since she had diabetes, she had to "move with a second person". She explained that "previously I was normal, I was Elizabeth free from diabetes, I could do anything without worry [...], but now I have another Elizabeth who worries about numbers, another Elizabeth whom I have to test and give insulin all the time and who can no longer sleep alone in the house because no one can help you in case of attack. It is a big responsibility but I accepted it."

Like Josh, Elizabeth is one of the few individuals I have met in Uganda, who had the possibility to own a glucometer and apply it regularly. Falling ill with diabetes means a break in one's life. A break from formerly being health to now having a chronic disease that will stay until death involving many moments of uncertainty. Especially when a person has to learn to classify bodily symptoms into the categories of high or low blood glucose levels, engaging in self-monitoring can be to regain confidence, as we have seen. For Elizabeth testing her glucose levels was a way to verify her feelings and foremost to keep death at a distance. The findings of the empirical part of this chapter will be discussed in more detail in the following section.

Numbers against uncertainty, numbers for a hopeful life

Numbers are important in various areas of our daily lives and may be used to express evidence of one sort or another: the body temperature to assess whether an individual has fever or not; the weight of an individual to assess if a person is obese, undernourished or just right; or measuring the blood sugar levels of a person with a glucometer to evaluate if a person has too high or too low glucose readings or if it is within the range. In the case of diabetes, it is the number that will identify an individual as being sick in the first place, and the number is not less important, when it comes to the monitoring of diabetes. The severity of the disease is expressed through a number; the success of the treatment is expressed through a number as well as individual conduct may be visualized with a number[23]. Also, an individual engaging in self-monitoring may express her- or himself, both bodily and emotionally, through a number. Though the numbers emerging from testing blood glucose levels may stand for one allegedly objective result, different people may attach different meanings or feelings to them, as this chapter intended to show. The numbers a glucometer produces, as Moretti (2016) states, "are elements socially built that do not offer a neutral worldview but, on the contrary, describe our reality while influencing whoever is using them. In this way numbers are not

---

23 Somewhat similar to other chronic diseases where regular testing identifies the general state of an individual. Just think of the CD4 cell count in HIV, blood pressure measurements etc.

[only] describing [a] reality but creating it".[24] How the numbers are created may vary according to who is intending to understand something or someone through them. The goal of self-monitoring is on the one hand to objectify the diabetic body through numbers. On the other hand, with the number individuals will gain more certainty and predictability about the disease, which is made visible, knowable and conveyable in shape of this number (cf. Guell 2009; 2012).

I have argued that the numbers arising from self-monitoring in the case of diabetes in Uganda cannot be detached from the device, the glucometer, with which they are generated and through which they become visible. The dual and ambivalent character of the device – limiting uncertainty and gaining more predictability about the disease while at the same time creating uncertainty in terms of the ability of maintaining the device economically and access wise – is inherent to the experience of testing and self-monitoring of diabetes in Uganda. In line with the argument I have developed in chapter five, the glucometer and the numbers it produces, may gain all the more meaning for the users the more its access and availability decreases against the backdrop of weak health infrastructures and limited (economical) resources. Self-monitoring is a practice, which cannot be taken for granted. A number then may gain ever more importance and reassurance due to the fact that it is not self-evident, and may have to serve and substitute for a long period of time.

As Nielsen and Grøn point out, the number produced through the glucometer appears not as static and fixed, but engaging in self-monitoring will signify an individual that they can have an impact on these numbers (Nielsen and Grøn 2013: 65). Continuous testing of glucose levels, as it is the case when a patient is involved in self-monitoring, creates fluid numbers due to the quantity and frequency of testing within one day (3-4 times as it was the case for Elizabeth and Josh). Fragmented testing on the contrary, as it is the case for most individuals who rely solely on governmental services, creates rather static and unchangeable numbers as they have to substitute for a much longer period (four weeks and more) until the next number will be produced. In this way numbers can become "inscription devices" the way Latour (1987) insinuated. Here, as Nielsen and Grøn state, "[t]he inscription quality of the numbers goes far beyond the biomedical domain when they work as phenomenological and moral devices that simultaneously reveal, reflect, and create experiences, emotions, and futures" (Nielsen and Grøn 2013: 70).

The narratives of Sister Joy, Josh and Elizabeth have shown that a glucometer indeed does more, means more and is used for more than merely measuring glucose levels and producing numbers. Engaging in the measurements of glucose levels utilizing a glucometer – even more so in the case of self-monitoring – can

---

24 https://easst.net/article/dealing-with-numbers-looking-beyond-the-self-monitoring-for-a-new-technology-of-the-self/.

be seen as an intervention to lock out one significant aspect that comes along with a chronic disease: uncertainty. When a person falls ill with a chronic disease, the well-known patterns and routines of everyday life have to yield and make way to a new life characterized by uncertainty and the need to redefine ones' self by ascribing new meaning to a new life situation. Using a glucometer and engaging in self-monitoring is one way of attributing this new meaning. The difference between contexts in the minority world and Uganda is the scarcity of technology, where testing the glucose level, respectively being tested by a medical professional, is not only a matter of choosing between testing and not testing, but a matter of practicability. A context where continuous testing often has to be replaced by scattered and fragmented testing, or not testing and being tested at all. Testing and self-monitoring here is not only a choice someone makes to engage in technologies of the self and enhance therapeutic outcomes, but relies on three cornerstones: The ability (how does the glucometer work and what do I need to know in order to use it?), the availability (do I have the testing strips and batteries to perform the test?) and the feasibility (the combination of ability and availability) of performing a test in the first place. This has important implications for the perception and understanding of self-monitoring and the compromise it often comes along with.

The point of departure of putting a glucometer to use differed between the three individuals in one simple but significant aspect: Sister Joy used one glucometer to test 418 patients, she was confronted with a situation of having to take care of 418 registered patients, knowing that only the minority of them was able to engage in self-monitoring to be better controlled "because they helped to control." It was her responsibility to prevent her patients from getting into a situation of medical complication and keeping her patients alive – by testing many of them only every second month, respectively on their coming to the health center. Elizabeth and Josh on the other hand each had one glucometer only for themselves. Elizabeth and Josh cannot be seen representative for the majority, but instead account for the minority of diabetes patients in Uganda. Nevertheless, we could see how continuous testing, respectively the meaning attached to the numbers emerging from this testing, can influence the perception of the disease. The disease becomes manageable, you can "monitor life", when the glucose levels are controlled on a regular basis and therefore the ability increases to see an immediate correlation between food and medication intake and exercise. Most importantly, when monitoring, one is able to keep death at a distance and stay alive as one may be able to act upon life threatening glucose levels. In this way, self-monitoring functioned not only as a gateway to the inner body, by visualizing glucose levels on the display, but further as a connector between the biomedical self and the emotional self.

Especially Josh mentioned how important it was for him to test in "order to know" himself. Mol points out for the case of diabetes patients in the Netherlands, that the glucometer "is [then] used in reaction to and as a correction of the feelings [this] may reach the point where such things as 'feelings' vanish behind the numbers" (Mol 2009: 15). My observations, however, showed that feelings did not necessarily disappear behind the numbers. On the contrary, they were produced and fostered by these numbers. Though regular testing could be perceived as an intruding aspect of the daily routines – like Mol (2009) observed – both, Elizabeth as well as Josh, felt "freedom" because they had access to their numbers whenever they felt bad. This in turn gave them the feeling of being able to "live a better life", a life beyond moments of uncertainty, yet suffering from a disease "that changes like weather", or where "the signs are sometimes the same when [the glucose level] is low and when it is high". Elizabeth expressed how the glucometer gave her "hope and safety not to die a mysterious death".

The stories of Elizabeth and Josh are examples for which impact a technological device can have not only in the management and control of disease, but also in relation to emotions. If the number displayed on the glucometer was good they felt good, if it was bad, it made them feel bad, frightened and consecutively the fear of dying increased. Emotions and the assessment of the physical condition were closely linked to the number that would appear on the glucometer. A good number, or "magical number" like Josh called it, induced happiness, pride and comfort. The number here functioned as a representation of the state in which the individuals found themselves, which they were not able to identify without. For Josh the glucometer was a tool for reassurance and window to the inside of his body for which reason there was a "psychological attachment to the number on the meter". Josh even spoke of getting a "diabetes burnout", a state referring to "good numbers day in day out [letting you forget that] you have to live a certain lifestyle". With the help of numbers, we can become more attentive and conscious of our bodies. Yet it is not only the fact of *possessing* a glucometer, but it might give you a feeling of being in control of a situation where your body has failed you and is everything other than under control. The glucometer may serve as a tool and reminder of having to live a certain lifestyle as any misconduct, eating the wrong foods or not taking medication, will immediately reflect in "bad numbers". Though it can get frustrating at times, when the sugar levels remain high or too low, it is at the same time a means for encouragement to engage in exercise when it the sugar level is too high, as a warning when it is too low, as well as a tool for rewarding oneself when the level has been stable. Sister Joy did not always trust the glucometers her patients were using because she did not know whether they kept them properly, which contradicts her endeavors to encourage her patients to self-monitor their glucose levels. She saw the reason for high glucose readings in the lack of self-monitoring instead of seeing the high levels of glucose as a result of (unfortunate) circumstances. The patients would not know how "they really feel" if they would not test themselves regularly. They would "not be safe" without testing.

The glucometer is a device to make visible, what would not be visible without it. "The glucometer performs magic. You cannot look into your body, but with the glucometer you can", like Josh said. Especially in situations where it is tricky to differentiate between the different symptoms that come along with too high/low blood sugar levels as they are at times confusing, may appear similar and are hard to differentiate without testing. While numbers seem to represent more objectivity than a subjective description of bodily symptoms would, it is important to keep in mind that "like words, numbers also can be evaluated in terms other than [...] as representations. Numbers that defy conventions or expectations can be infelicitous as well as wrong" (Espeland and Stevens 2008: 403).

In this chapter I aimed to show that a glucometer and the numbers it produces can be the vehicle and tool for a redefinition and a way of repairing and giving sense to a ruptured life caused by disease. Disruptions in life are unavoidable. Human experience is generally characterized by uncertainty. However, in chronic diseases uncertainty becomes an even more menacing danger, because it persists. Maynard states, "although continuity in life is an elusive narrative, it is an effective one" (Maynard 2010: 195) since it orders and organizes peoples' trajectories and expectations in life and how we come to understand who we are and what we do. Self-monitoring, though its usefulness is contested, is a desired practice and can be seen as one way of restoring and maintaining continuity, with the use of the glucometer and the making of numbers.

7. Seek and you shall find: Medical Outreaches

> Seeking what is true
> is not seeking what is desirable
> ——Albert Camus 1955: 41

"You know," Ismael, the assistant of the district health officer said, "diagnostics are one essential part in the whole chaos of our health care system, yet the given structure here in Uganda is often preventing it [...]. We have many actions going on for HIV here in this country with projects, campaigns and outreaches. For diabetes it is a problem, it is hard to start an initiative if there is no money from the government. And international organizations are not interested to invest money. These projects, no matter for which disease, are also a problem. Even if it seems good that they are here, one day the international organizations will leave, but we will stay. Without drugs and equipment, you cannot deal with disease properly."

Three aspects become apparent in Ismael's quote, which will serve to mark the course this chapter shall pursue: firstly, diagnostics and testing for disease play a major role within any health care system. As already described in chapter five, it is the moment, when a disease gets a name and blurry symptoms receive an explanation. Further it is the moment, when alleged clarity and certainty sets in and, in the best case, curative treatment can be brought on the way. Chapter five has nevertheless shown that, while a diagnostic act may be an order making tool, it can at the same time create disorder in the lives of the diagnosed, especially in chronic conditions, where there is no cure and long-term care needs to be provided. Therefore, a diagnosis may bring clarity and relief while it can come along with confusion and dread simultaneously. Secondly, also recalling chapter three, without a functioning and stable health infrastructure that includes "stuff, staff and space" (Farmer 2014; Street 2014c), as well as the necessary knowledge to approach and handle a disease, a diagnostic act may not only become a difficult undertaking. But, once performed, may cause an already fragile health care system to overexert even more, respectively it may not be capable of providing the needed care. As Smith-Morris put it "diagnosis must be the gateway to an organized system of treatment" (Smith-Morris 2016: 20). Testing followed by a diagnosis is only a first step, but there have to be infrastructures in place to provide the needed care and keep it going, especially in chronic diseases. Finally, the Ugandan health care system (and others of the majority world) is largely shaped by what Ismael calls "projects, campaigns and outreaches". This is what Whyte et al. (2013) refer to as a "projectified landscape of care", which is highly shaped by and dependent on international aid projects. This is the case especially for HIV/AIDS and other communicable diseases (Whyte 2013; see also Biehl and Petryna 2013 and DelVecchio Good), Good, and Grayman 2010). This chapter will touch upon each of these aspects, but perhaps not in the way you may anticipate.

The diagnostic act we will encounter in this chapter is an effort by different actors to make diabetes visible in individuals and communities. Because one way of diagnosing people with diabetes is not by waiting until they come to the health centers (when the disease is in a progressed state), but to go for medical outreaches[1]. Instead engaging in community screening practices is a possibility "to bring the clinic to the villages and grab the disease in its beginnings", as a health worker once described. In fact, outreaches and screening practices are a common and often welcomed way of uncovering disease before an individual has experienced any kind of unusual and disturbing bodily sensation. It is a way of uncovering disease at a state, in which it is not anticipated by showing itself through clear signs and symptoms.[2] Jutel, referring to an article by Armstrong (1995), describes screening as a means to reveal illness before an individual has experienced any kind of symptom (Jutel 2011: 126; see also Han 1997; Lupton 1995; 2001). She states that in screening

---

1 "To go for an outreach" was the designation that was used in Uganda to refer to screening practices outside the hospital setting within a community and will be used interchangeably with screening practices throughout this chapter.
2 David Armstrong (1995) describes the evolvement from "bedside medicine" – where the doctor came to patient's homes, relying on the individual description of symptoms by the patients themselves – to "hospital medicine" at the end of the 18th century, situated in a hospital "where the focus is less on patients identified symptoms, but on signs detected by the doctor and laboratory tests performed by the medical staff" (Armstrong 1995: 393). During the 20th century, rather than looking for disease merely inside an individual's body, disease was likewise located outside the body as a germinating potential within a whole population. Armstrong designates this as "surveillance medicine" that sees diseases perpetually hovering within and between humans and can be managed by screening allegedly healthy populations (ibid.). One of the effects of surveillance medicine, namely that an individual should and can engage (or gets engaged) in intermittent health investigations even when feeling well or, put differently, even though not experiencing any signs and symptoms that could hint at an underlying disease, is by no means new. In fact, already in the mid-nineteenth century the physician Horace Dobell argued that a disease is heralded by "pre-existent physiological states of 'low health'" followed by the assumption that therapies show more effect at an earlier stage of disease. Intermittent health investigations would therefore be a way of identifying "these earliest evasive periods of defect in the physiological state, and to adopt measures for their remedy" (Dobell 1861 in Han 1997: 910).

"symptoms are not coterminous with disease. Rather, disease is seen as a silent, unobtrusive potentiality, ready to rear its ugly head in the seemingly healthy when least expected" (ibid.: 127). Where medicinal practices are usually applied *after* a disease has occurred or *while* it is still occurring, screening "extends the diagnostic power to a space *before* disease" (Jutel 2011: 127, emphasis in the original. See also Armstrong 1995). Prominent examples are screening programs for breast cancer or cancer of the cervix. The message transported is simple: participate in a screening program and the likelihood that you will fall victim to a disease is minimized. Hopes will be fueled that the earlier for instance cancer is found, the better the prospects of either not falling ill at all or of regaining full recovery in case the disease is found early (ibid.; see also Smith-Morris 2016: 148).

Especially the new global health and its push for medical technologies has fostered the use of point-of-care devices for such undertakings that are not bound and fixed to a certain place and are easy to use. Medical examinations are then not necessarily dependent on hospitals or doctors' offices that have laboratories. With this the scope and therefore the number of individuals reached with screening practices expands. Screening can now take place for instance in a primary school of a village; on a piece of abandoned agricultural land underneath temporarily pitched tents; in a small pharmacy or at the busy roadside of a main road connecting the east and the central region of Uganda. Locations we will find ourselves in in the following empirical vignettes. We will enter different settings, where different actors with different intentions, different knowledges, backgrounds, and different monetary preconditions. We will see how diabetes (and other diseases) can be uncovered outside the conventional biomedical setting: endeavors by a Ugandan health facility to extend the clinic and screen people in circumjacent communities; outreaches conducted by a group of North Americans as an "educational practice"; finally, the attempts of a private sports health club to take over the responsibility, where it is perceived that the government has failed to fulfill its obligations. Though the premises and objectives differ between these three actors, they yet all want to reach one goal: identify individuals suffering from diabetes before they themselves know.

The three different projects or efforts offering diabetes testing are not initiated by large health organizations or supported by large donor funds like for infectious diseases. However, I propose to read the empirical vignettes as a form of what Wendland (2010) refers to as "resourcefulness – the capacity to secure any available tools, equipment, social networks, and funds" (ibid.: 173) for a condition like diabetes that has been neglected. Taking the chance to use the resources when – as in the following examples – foreigners come to help or individuals in Uganda have mobilized funds, can on the one hand be seen as a way to substitute and complement a weak health infrastructure. On the other hand – and to hark back to the overarching question of this work, how diabetes is made visible and understandable in a health care system that has mostly dealt with infectious diseases in the past – I suggest that the efforts we will encounter in this chapter are a way of 'doing good' by contributing to make diabetes visible, heard, and knowable. The act of diagnosing hereby is not only a way of uncovering diabetes, but can further be understood as a way of granting access to diagnostic tools as part of a humanitarian and altruistic endeavor. The Ugandan health care system is characterized by a weak health infrastructure, with lack of access to diagnostics and treatment for diabetes. This lack or incompleteness may, however, supposedly be turned into an opportunity by individuals who seek to fill this incompleteness or gap with action. Or, to say it with the words of Wendland (2010) nudge a shift "from a problem into an opportunity" (Wendland 2010: 174). A logic of chance, if you want (see chapter five).

The new global health that has emerged from its older 'sister' international health[3], does not only operate in a global health world within in which the reliance and strive for metrics, measurability and evidence seems to dictate the global health agendas and with this the prioritization of diseases. It further operates within two main poles: "a register of protection, in which its primary focus is international health security, and within a register of compassionate aid, in which it concerns itself foremost with the alleviation of suffering and health inequalities" (Crane 2013: 152). In short: the new global health may well be positioned at the interface of global health security and humanitarian biomedicine (Lakoff 2010; Cohen 2006; see also chapter two). What, however, does this mean for a chronic disease like diabetes, which, as I have stated before, may not fit well in either of these two regimes of global health? It can neither be framed as a threat for the health security in the sense that it spreads across borders putting the lives of the global public at risk, nor has it up to date become a prominent subject and endeavor of humanitarian aid.

Redfield (2008) suggests that once a disease or a disaster in general is framed as a humanitarian emergency, it provokes calls for action and "the affected communities and those experiencing anguish secondhand through the wonders of global media commonly expect response" (Redfield 2008: 147). Likewise, Street (2014c) states that as soon as the disease burden of a fragile state is termed as a 'crisis' "the case is made for immediate action that draws attention away from state building and 'good governance' and toward the need to save as many lives as is possible with as little money in the least amount of time" (Street 2014c: 227f.). Lakoff and Collier (2008) reason that organizations in the field of global health are gravitated to states of emergency because they "galvanize public attention and resources in a way that long-term problems do not. Another [reason] is that – at least from the vantage of first-order actors – measures focused on mitigating potential emergencies are

---

3 Whether it actually differs in its approaches and is distinct from each other is debated (Crane 2013: 152).

easier to implement than longer-term structural interventions" (ibid.: 17). Indeed, the problem with chronic diseases is that they do not "break out" like infectious diseases do, implying a state of emergency, which requires immediate re-action to halt the spread within and between nations. What they do is they "creep up" (Bury 1982: 170; see also chapter five) and may lurk in the bodies of individuals often unnoticed until they strike. There are no quick fixes for chronic diseases, neither are there magic bullets or "technological 'silver bullet' solutions, such as pharmaceuticals, mosquito nets, or rapid diagnostic tests" (Street 2014c: 227f.). Once a chronic disease has been diagnosed, it will be and stay present until death.

The image motif of the picture we can paint in this 21st century seems quite clear: the new global health has been followed by a considerable upsurge in funding for infectious diseases, not for chronic diseases. International health agencies such as the World Health Organization are putting an emphasis on disease control to be prepared for potential outbreaks of infectious diseases (Street 2014c; Crane 2013). Philanthropic organizations like the Bill and Melinda Gates Foundation made it their business to cope with global health threats by working on and implementing low-cost interventions mostly for HIV and malaria (Lakoff and Collier 2008: 17). Humanitarian organizations such as *Médicins Sans Frontières* (Doctors without Borders) draw their motivation from the reduction of human suffering and death in contexts of urgent emergencies (ibid.; Redfield 2012a and 2013). Global health interventions of all kinds, by different actors with various ambitions and different preconditions aim to bring humanitarian aid to underserved and under-resourced countries. They seek to act in the "name of human rights development" (Wendland 2010: 9) and in the name of "humanitarianism, development and security" (Biehl and Petryna 2013: 6; see also Fassin 2012b; Lakoff and Collier 2008).

As a consequence of the inflation of humanitarian aid projects much of the basic health care services have been outsourced to non-governmental and non-state organizations. What is termed "health system strengthening" can be put on a level with public-private 'partnership', which paradoxically "leads to the further fragmentation of health into a series of 'projects' run by different organizations, further depleting the public spaces and systems that exist at their interstices" (Street 2014c: 229; Whyte 2013). State of the art health facilities especially for HIV/AIDS where "wealthy donors create showcase clinics", equipped with high-tech technology, then exist side by side with decayed governmental health facilities (Biehl and Petryna 2013: 135). Settings with weak health infrastructures and fragile health care systems, limited access to diagnostic tests and pharmaceuticals seem to offer a great 'playground' for gaining new experience and learning what it means and takes to "do global health". Where, as we will see in one of the following empirical vignettes "we get to do a lot of things we are not allowed to do in the US". Spaces, where it seems that 'good' can be done, yet also spaces with "easy access to patient bodies" (Crane 2013: 169). It is these settings, where individuals want to travel to as volunteers or "clinical tourists"[4] to "do good" in a short-term assignment.

In her beautiful and attentive ethnography, Wendland (2010; 2012) offers insights to clinical tourists from North America who are seeking to extend their (medical) experience in a Malawian hospital. The encounter between Malawian doctors and northern American medical students "troubled them [the Malawian doctors], enhancing their awareness of the contradiction between their high status, product of a globalized idea of the doctor, and the realities of their day-to-day work, firmly lodged with the poverty-stricken South" (Wendland 2010: 218). The question therefore may indeed be posed, who the beneficiaries are at the end of the day, when "they will leave, but we will stay", like the quote from Ismael stated above (see also Crump and Sugarman 2008; Crane 2013: 169). This question may especially be posed in this chapter, where some of the volunteers we will come to meet, are not even medical students or have anything to do with medicine. Instead their experiences are made in the minority world and their medicinal knowledge is limited to taking body temperature. As what kind of "doing good" can such an endeavor be understood?

Volunteerism or voluntary work, "the free giving of an individual's labor, time, and energy to a larger cause, collective goal, or public good"[5] (Brown and Prince 2015: 29; cf. Eliasoph 2011; Redfield & Bornstein 2010), has become a popular. It is a way of being committed to and get involved in development, humanitarian and philanthropic activities and activisms with the provision of health care increasingly standing at its core (ibid.; cf. Milligan and Conradson 2006; Abramowitz and Panter-Brick 2015). It insinuates the formation or "enactment of attachment between the individual and a collective and carries assumptions about altruism, freedom, and a 'politics of virtue' (ibid; cf. Mindry 2001). It is what Brown and Prince (2015) refer to as a "powerful concept, capable of mobilizing individuals and groups to act for a common good" (ibid.: 30). As Brown and Prince (2015) continue:

> While volunteering is a global phenomenon, it is also situated within historically specific political and economic contexts. Assumptions about altruistic action, freedom, and virtue that surround the concept do not therefore necessarily hold. Despite such ideals, the actual practice of volunteering is often riddled with

---

[4] Following Wendland (2010; 2012) a clinical tourist can be defined as an individual travelling to a foreign country, mostly to a country in the minority world, to exchange medical goods and ideas. I is often assumed that "the Northern institution has not just the financial but the intellectual capital, while the Southern institution has the raw materials (including exotic patients and pathogens) ready to be extracted (Wendland 2010: 291; emphasis in the original).

[5] Or it may be framed as "encounters between privilege and poverty" (Muehlebach 2012ad: 300; see also Mindry 2001; Redfield & Bornstein 2010; see also Redfield 2012b).

tension. Volunteering may benefit the giver as much as the receiver. The lines between altruism and material reward, and between labor that is given freely and labor that is demanded by those in political authority, are often blurred. The relation between voluntary labor and paid work may be ambiguous, and the utility of volunteering within the labor market may be significant. Although imagined as progressive social action, voluntary labor as charitable, humanitarian, or development practice may reinforce inequalities between giver and recipient. (ibid. 2015: 30; cf. Mittermaier 2014)

This chapter intends to extend the gaze of conventional notions of clinical tourism and volunteerism and includes not only the 'doing good' by foreign individuals, traveling thousands of kilometers to help the 'underserved'. Further it sheds light on the 'doing good from *within*' by Ugandan individuals who see it as their obligation to do what the government and international organizations seem to fail in doing. The 'doing good from within' seems to be independent of the ideals of the global health humanitarianism, independent of the world of metrics, which make these actions possible in the first place. It is a form of humanitarianism, which can set in when exactly these measures and efforts are few. It is a field, which opens up, which draws its justification from the alleged lack of governmental and international action to combat a specific disease.

Yet there are dangers in a diagnostic screening tests, especially when it is not embedded in a permanent and formalized health care system, but takes place rather uncoordinatedly. The raising of false hopes for example, especially when they are actually not part of the regular health care practices and only take place randomly and often only once. It is then when what has started out as an endeavor to shift a problem into an opportunity like Wendland (2010) had it in mind, may create a new problem. Shifting the problem of a lacking access to diabetes diagnostics in Uganda into the opportunity of granting this access outside the average health care system. Yet the problem of rising numbers of individuals with diabetes has to be tackled exactly within the average health care system. A diagnosis alone is not enough, but access to continuous testing as well as pharmaceutical treatment have to follow. What has started out as efforts to strengthen a health care system, may shift in weakening it even more. This chapter will take us to different settings where testing and diagnostic practices for diabetes and other diseases takes place outside the conventional health care system. The following will describe a snapshot of an outreach undertaken by a laboratory technician of a governmental health center. What had previously started as a larger program in Uganda, the 'Family Health Days', to increase the reach of medical services in the communities, is now nothing more than a remainder.

The crowd pullers

Like almost every Tuesday, I arrived at the health center in district X at around 9 a.m. The laboratory had opened its doors, it had been cleaned and everything that would be needed for the day was prepared. The waiting area was rapidly filling up with people who had come to be tested. Some of them would be tested for malaria, some for HIV. Others would have to give a urine sample or a blood sample and again others would be tested for diabetes. However, it was one of these mornings, where the glucometer would be taken away from the laboratory to another place, together with a vial of 25 testing strips, a package of HIV testing kits including 100 tests, and around 50 malaria Rapid Diagnostic testing kits (RDTs). Eric, one of the laboratory technicians, put all these things, alongside his medical scrubs, in a box. "Today" he said, "you and I will go for an outreach". He told me that once in a while he would go to nearby trading centers to screen people. Before we left the health center to head to the testing site, Eric collected a few pharmaceuticals from the dispensary: some painkillers as well as some deworming tablets, which would be given to children. A health worker came along as well, who would be responsible for distributing condoms and giving advice on matters of maternal health and family health planning. In irregular intervals a trading center close to the facility was chosen and outreaches were conducted for a couple of hours in the morning. This time in a trading center about 2 km away. Eric did not know whose idea or order this undertaking really was, but "that's just what we do sometimes", he said. Later I would come to understand, that this was a remnant of a program that had been initiated between UNICEF and the Ministry of Health, the so-called Family Health Days, which we will get back to shortly.

It was almost 10 a.m. when we arrived at a pharmacy that also was a bakery and would function as the testing site for the next four hours. I helped Eric prepare a small bench, a small table and a chair for the person to be tested in front of the pharmacy. It was smelling like cake and pastries mixed with a touch of freshly fried samosas. I asked Eric whether the people around even knew that he was here to offer free testing or how else would they know what was going on? But there was no need for an announcement, "you will see, the people will come", he assured. Indeed, it did not take long until the first person came and the testing started. Compared to the other outreaches I joined, this one – with one laboratory technician and a health worker – was a lot smaller in its scope, but also a lot more personal. Eric as well as the health worker had time for the individuals and could answer all sorts of questions. They also knew some of the people. Young boys and adolescents provoked laughter once in a while when they came to collect condoms, commenting with phrases such as "you give me more than this, I need many".

It was a Tuesday morning, a weekday. The people who came were tested en passant, in between their obligations and everyday business. Some were carrying their groceries; some bodaboda[6] drivers stopped "let me take a test", before they would continue to transport their passengers to their destinations. Five people had been tested for diabetes so far, none of them had any abnormalities in their glucose levels. "The good thing about this kind of testing", Eric explained, while we were waiting for the next person to come for testing "it is a kind of testing we can do on the roadside, and it made us capture many patients. Many people who did not know they were sick. Like for DM [diabetes mellitus], the testing has brought many more patients with DM now. They all wouldn't have known without it."

Though the testing was perceived to be a good practice, some of the statements I heard from individuals who came to be tested that day reflected a fear of the testing, respectively fear of the test result. One woman who wanted to be tested, pulled her finger back before the needle could prick her finger to draw blood for the glucose test. It was, however, not the fear of the needle, she feared that the result would "turn out positive". She said "for me I feel that I want to know if it [diabetes] is there. But I fear it too much. I have an aunty who died of diabetes this year. I do not know what I would do if it is positive. Maybe it is better I do not know." In the end, the woman left without testing her glucose levels. Another tested person explained that testing for disease is never easy. Especially if it is a disease like diabetes: "This sukali [diabetes] is very bad. It can kill you fast and it makes you suffer." Yet another aspect came up during the forenoon: people kept on thanking Eric not only for coming to their village, but for sparing them from having to go to the health center where "we wait so long" or "they get rude and unfriendly" or "they do not have time for you". Indeed, the testing had somewhat of a testing with an easy atmosphere, a testing en passant with a good feeling attached to it, rather than waiting to be tested at a health center when feeling sick and weak.

The glucose testing was abruptly interrupted when a lady came to be tested for diabetes – after the usual procedure of drawing blood, applying it onto the strip and inserting the strip into the glucometer. The device showed and error. "Error 5" was indicated on the screen. Eric tried again several times, each time using a new testing strip, but the glucometer failed to produce a result. Eric did not know what Error 5 meant. "Usually when the meter fails to work, I switch it off and turn it on again and then it works. But this time I think it is now dead". Later we figured out that Error 5 denoted that the glucometer needed cleansing.[7] But for that day, there would not be any further diabetes testing available. People who wanted to be tested for 'sukali' would have to relinquish and wait for the next opportunity.

---

6 A bodaboda is a motorcycle taxi and an important means of transport in the villages in Uganda.
7 The glucometer Eric was using was an old brand, where the drop of blood was applied directly onto the strip and inserted into the machine, meaning that there were always some residues left in the machine. The newer machines use testing strips where the blood is not inserted directly into the machine (see chapter four of this book).

One week had passed since the outreach with Eric in the pharmacy. It was only by coincidence that I came across the Family Health Days. I was on my way to the grocery store to buy some water when passing by a building with a big banner stretched across. At first sight I did not think about it too much, how could I have known that these Family Health Days were connected to the outreach that had taken place a week before? I found out in a meeting with the district health officer (DHO) of district X that the Family Health Days were developed as a tool to accelerate positive outcomes especially related to the Millennium Development Goals (MDGs) 4 "Reduce Child Mortality" and MDG 5 "Improve Maternal Health". When the Ugandan Ministry of Health and UNICEF recognized a stagnation in achieving the Millennium Development Goals, they together commenced the so-called "Family Health Days" in 2012. One of the responsible employees of UNICEF Uganda, Dr. K., explained to me that

> "the biggest killers in relation to children in Uganda, or sub-Saharan Africa for that matter, are diarrhea and upper respiratory tract infections and malaria. We sat together and were brainstorming what we can do. Against pneumonia we have this vaccine[8], which was introduced already and it is working. We have iCCM, the integrated community case management[9], which focuses on these three. But the effects were stagnating and we were thinking what should we do in order to help accelerate the MDGs?"

Before the Family Health Days there was a program, "Child Days Plus", specifically designed to target children. As Dr. K. put it, it the actions during Child Day Plus were "reduced to distributing Vitamin A and deworming tablets to children". They discovered that in April and October, when the Child Day Plus were taking place, there was a peak in immunization. They thought that if Child Day Plus was successful in relation to the immunization coverage, "why don't we have four peaks if we do another program in addition, support the routine services by extending its reach, identifying low-coverage areas where the routine services are not enough", Dr. K. deduced. That is how the idea of the Family Health Days was born in January 2012 and was implemented six months later.

I was starting to wonder how glucose testing and testing for hypertension were related to this undertaking. Dr. K. explained that the reason why they called it Family Health Days was standing to reason, as compared to the Child Days Plus the new program intended to actively involve the parents of the children. By offering free

---

8 The vaccine is abbreviated with PCV and stands for Pneumococcal Conjugate Vaccine.
9 The Integrated Community Case Management (iCCM) is a strategy by the Ministry of Health of Uganda to extend its reach of the public health services in remote areas, by providing treatment for malaria, pneumonia and diarrhea especially to infants under the age of five (see WHO 2016b, http://www.who.int/malaria/areas/community_case_management/overview/en/).

blood pressure testing and, in case of a high blood pressure, additional testing for diabetes. The supply section from UNICEF decided which devices to purchase based primarily on the costs. They provided all the supplies, including the glucometers, the blood pressure machines, data collection materials such as tally-sheets. For antenatal care they provided examination beds, stethoscopes, phonoscopes and so on. UNICEF, however, did not cater for the glucometer testing strips. It was the Ministry of Health of Uganda that was responsible for the provision of the testing strips, mainly due to the fact that UNICEF is not mandated to provide care to people above the age of 45.

To include screening for hypertension and diabetes, though the focus of UNICEF is on children, was based on an effort from the Ministry of Health of Uganda to "spread the possibilities of revealing these tricky diseases. This way we kill two birds with one stone". Offering testing for the parents of the children had "a really intelligent idea behind it, because the involvement of men in this patriarchal society encourages also mothers to come. Often men have to give permission, or are the ones who give money for transport." What became obvious quite fast was that the blood pressure testing as well as the glucose testing were crowd pullers, a magnet to attract masses of people. "In some places, there were crowds because people wanted to test their blood pressure and their sugar levels", Dr. K. remembered.

The spatial alignment was distinct from the outreaches I would be attending later on, which will be described in the following. The UNICEF and the Ministry of Health came up with the idea to use a different platform than where outreaches often take place, such as schools. They figured out that the coverage at religious facilities, that is places of worship, was 45-times higher than the coverage of health facilities and that the religious leaders were furthermore people who were highly respected and trusted, as an employee of the Ministry of Health reasoned in an interview. Further

> "they are capable of mobilizing people. These are already existing structures, which do not need any investment and they are also recognizable. Where this and that church is, everybody knows and they are close to the people as well, that is one thing. Then the next thing is that 90% of the Ugandan population worship and they go to churches or mosques. We wanted to use that availability. We know that what is really preventing people from taking services is the opportunity associated with it. Because of the proximity to places of worship, and when you have a table next to the place when they come out, you take that opportunity, right?"

After some time, they sat together to evaluate the effectiveness of the program. It became clear that there was "a lot of resistance from the Ministry [of Health of Uganda] of who said we were installing something parallel [to the available governmental health services] and taking too much attention and killing the routine service", as a member of the Ministry of Health of Uganda explained. Other voices got loud, stressing the cumbersomeness and expenses of this undertaking. With the help of an external evaluation company they concluded that the services offered were useful, that antenatal care as well as offering glucose testing, however, should be withdrawn from the program as it was "too complicated". Despite the recommendations to end the screening for hypertension and diabetes, the Ministry of Health wished to continue especially with the blood sugar screening. As I was told by Dr. K.

> "they wanted to have it as a public health measure, screening these people and referring them to care. That was the idea. But the resources limited them and they could not pack it up with resources. We give tetanus vaccine to young girls and women in a reproductive age from 15-45. That makes sense because if you take a look at the continuum of care, if the mother is in good shape, the child is probably in good shape. Why we included blood pressure and glucose screening is because the Ministry of Health of Uganda wanted to use the platform. We could not say no, because of course we also hear about the increased numbers of these chronic diseases. I like it as a public health person. But there is a limit to how much you can stretch yourself because you also need to justify it towards your money providers. How could we do that? It is a problem."

There were positive outcomes especially concerning the coverage and also the acceptance of the program. Further it was one of the first attempts to generate data on diabetes and hypertension. "Before that there was not really any centered blood sugar or diabetes screening. It was the first data that we had. Before it was nearly zero". Yet the program ended in October 2014 and was continued as the "Integrated Child Health Days" afterwards – without screening for diabetes. Dr. K. was disappointed that a good idea "was killed" because of lacking resources. However, as we have seen, it was not fully killed, Eric continued to offer screening with the possibilities he had at hand.

Dr. K. shared some of his doubts about outreach and screening programs such as the Family Health Days: how could telling people they may have hypertension or diabetes on the one hand and not providing services on the other be justified? What would happen with all those individuals after they were told they might suffer from such a disease? As he put it: "You screen them somewhere on the roadside and then what do you do after that? It is not only about screening but also about the capacity of the health care system to deliver the required services. You wonder if it is good to know and die or you do not know and die? I don't know. Unless you deliver that service, it is not enough to just screen. As a public health person, you need to keep that in mind too."

This section described outreach efforts as the leftover the Family Health Days. With the intention to increase the degree of the immunization of children, glucose testing and blood pressure measuring was offered as well to attract more people. Spaces of worship, so the assumption, offer a suitable space to get hold of many people. The outreach I described in the beginning was, however, a lot smaller in scope and the equipment used for this purpose was not any longer provided by UNICEF, but was the equipment from the governmental health center IV in district X. The glucometer that served for the testing was, for the time of the outreach, unavailable at the health center. Yet these efforts, like Eric explained, were important because it made him capture many individuals with diabetes who did not know they were suffering from the disease before. That the glucometer broke, respectively had an error which could not be rectified on site, led to an abrupt termination of the efforts. The next section will bring us to the roadside of a suburb of Kampala. 'Bo-Health-Club', a sports club in Kampala, took the action and initiated one day of community outreach as an act of altruism and endeavor to substitute for the perceived lack of governmental actions to combat diabetes. A lack of functioning technology will not be a problem in this example.

"An act of giving without receiving"

I was on my way to the health center IV in district X again. How many times now had I left Kampala before to head there? Certainly, I could dream the way, I would have to pass several roundabouts on my way out of Kampala, with a traffic jam before one of the larger roundabouts nearly every morning. It was a roundabout next to a market, where various goods were sold. Fish, fruit, meat, vegetables and the like. Bicycles, bodabodas, trucks, cars, pedestrians – all trying to find a way either into or out of the roundabout to continue their way. Street vendors took the chance, peddling their goods through open car windows, offering water or sodas against the thirst, nuts and cookies against the small hunger, chewing gum and lots of other things. As the major road connecting the East and the West of Uganda, this roundabout was a bottleneck for anybody who wanted to leave or enter Uganda's capital city via this route, especially in the morning or evening hours. Sitting in my car, a bit annoyed due to the slow-moving traffic, I listened to some cheerful tunes a friend of mine had pulled on a thumb drive for me. I opened the windows, to let the small breeze float inside one window for it to exit from the other.

It was only one last roundabout before I would have to take a turn left to stay on the main road and take course towards the health center, a fifteen minutes' drive (if there was no traffic jam), passing several petrol stations and three trading centers. Though it was a Saturday morning, the traffic was very busy and therefore I moved forward only very slowly. This nevertheless gave me the time to look around and observe. Perhaps if the traffic would not have been as busy this morning, I would not have noticed the loud music coming from the other side of the road, which drew my attention. My eyes went rightwards and caught sight of a white pavilion, a lot of people standing around it and a big banner "Free diabetes checking and counseling". It took only a few seconds for me to reorganize my schedule for the day. The health center could wait, I thought. Determined to figure out what was happening here by the roadside I parked the car. The trading center was stuffed with people and vehicles, I was lucky to find a small space in front of a supermarket – I approached the pavilion. Four health workers – I assumed they were health workers for they were all wearing white medical scrubs – were sitting at a table covered with a colorful table cloth, three were testing, one was writing into a book. I counted two glucometers as well as some HIV tests, which were lying on the table. A queue of about fifteen people had lined up for the testing. Behind the tent there were some chairs, where a health worker was taking blood pressure measurements.

A young woman, who would later introduce herself as Grace, came up to me with a huge and welcoming smile on her face. She was wearing a sports dress: shorts, a Polo-Shirt and sneakers, as if she was ready to go for a run. We started a conversation, exchanging information and thoughts. She told me that it was the first time they were offering this kind of testing. She herself came from Bo-Health Club, a sports club composed of people, who met and worked out together to "improve their health", as she explained. She invited me to stay at the testing site and join in what was happening, clearly excited that I was, too, working on diabetes: "This is good, we need as many people working on it [diabetes] as possible." The music in the background, which was coming from big speakers behind the tent, seemed to spread good vibes. All people appeared to be cheerful and happy, some were moving with the beat, one woman was singing along.

The testing ran under the slogan "Diabetes can be prevented". As I had seen before, additional testing for HIV and high blood pressure was offered, "as a bonus", as Grace explained. The testing team itself comprised four health workers and a doctor from a nearby governmental health center. Five members of Bo-Health Club, without a medical background, assisted in the testing and oversaw the actions. They also took care of the people coming for the testing, making sure they were lining up correctly and ready to give information about the health club, encouraging the people to become part of the club and do more sports. A team mixed with professionals and non-professionals working together to make the testing possible: the professionals provided their medical and technical knowledge and the non-medical professionals had provided the equipment – glucometers and HIV rapid tests – and made sure that everyone felt comfortable. The people could decide themselves whether they wanted to be tested for all three diseases, or if they only wanted to be tested for certain diseases. One man who was standing in line was asking me "they are testing here for what?"

It became clear that not all people who came for the testing had the initial intention to be tested for diabetes because they simply did not yet know why the team was here and what was really happening. I asked a woman who was standing in line why she was here, and she answered "I just came and saw all those people standing here and now I want to test for HIV. I have in total tested four times for HIV and was always without HIV. But now I again want to know my status and also test for diabetes because I want to delete possibilities of disease." The man behind her added "I only want to test for diabetes since I already know my HIV status." When the patients had finished the testing, they were able to talk to a doctor, Dr. M., who was the in-charge of a nearby governmental health center III, in order to discuss the results and counsel the people who needed medical advice or referral. He was also the one to clarify the test results especially of the diabetes testing. "What does this mean here? I have diabetes or what?", a woman asked me, showing her test result, a number, written on a sheet of paper. Unlike tests that produce either a positive or a negative result, the glucometer does not indicate "positive" or "negative", but, as we have seen in the previous chapters, a number that requires interpretation. For the people who wanted to be tested, this number raised irritation and confusion of what it really meant and what to make of it. A "positive" or "negative" result was a lot easier to grasp, for it was clear that it meant the disease is either there, or it is not there. Instead the number that was written on the small piece of paper had no real use until someone had the time to explain this number. The number would then be translated in terms of a "good" or a "bad" result, or close to bad or still ok, but requiring actions taken to prevent it from becoming bad. This is clearly a difference to the tests they were used. Malaria, HIV or syphilis or other diseases, which could be tested with point-of-care devices indicated "positive" or "negative". The number a glucometer produces, however, requires the knowledge to categorize it according to the standards. The test results from an RDT in turn can be read by anybody who has understood that two bars indicate a positive testing result and one bar a negative result, which can be quickly grasped without much explanation and considering the fact that individuals are often not only tested once for malaria in their life. Sometimes, when a person received her result, she clearly had question marks in her eyes not knowing what to make of the number on her sheet. In such cases the team from Bo-Health Club took care of her, involving her in a conversation for instance on the activities of the sports club until the doctor had time to discuss the result with her. Everything seemed to go smooth and hand in hand.

Grace told me that compared to HIV testing that often came along with shame and people preferred to test "in quiet places", people were excited to be tested for diabetes. "Some of them even asked when we are coming back", she told me. She said that people wanted to tell their family and friends who had missed the opportunity to test that day. Everybody knew someone with diabetes "and it is now a disease we all fear that is why we want to test to know". The numbers of tests performed for HIV and diabetes reflected her statement. While the number of people tested for HIV was limited to a few, the number of people who wanted to be tested for diabetes were many. One-hundred-and-forty tests were performed with the glucometer compared to around 30 tests for HIV that day. Nevertheless, some people I asked what they wanted to test for and why answered that they wanted to be tested for diabetes as they already knew their HIV status. All the tests performed were recorded in the health centers outpatient book, which would then be transferred to the weekly HMIS[10] data registration system. The data of the diabetes testing was additionally entered into a small booklet, which would stay with Dr. M. as a synopsis. Of the 140 tests that had been performed that day, six individuals had an elevated blood sugar. Dr. M. told me that they used a cut-off value for an elevated blood sugar at 130 mg/dL [7,2 mmol/L][11]. Any individual who had a level above this value, would be asked if she had eaten or not before the test (as food increases the blood sugar level) and given advice on diet. In case the individual had not eaten before the test and their glucose levels exceeded 130 mg/dL, Dr. M. instructed them to come to his health center the following week to repeat the test. "I could not give a diagnosis based only on one test", Dr. M. said.

I wanted to know more about how this Bo-Health Club and how the idea to test for diabetes on the roadside had arisen. It was the first time I had seen something like this and I was admittedly excited. I exchanged details with Grace and Dr. M. so that we could meet another day, when there was a bit more time and quietness. This is how I met Grace again a few days later. Filled with pride and excitement she told me that Bo-Health Club already started back in 2007. It would not be common in Uganda that people do sports, she told me. A man came up with the idea to initiate a club like this because he was suffering from hypertension and his doctor recommended him to engage in physical activities in order to keep his blood pressure low. When he started with his training, he started thinking that he surely was not the only person suffering from hypertension. The idea behind the club was to bring people who were exercising alone together so that exercising could be an act of togetherness and a shared effort. "It is not good for everybody to do their own thing, but it is good to collect ourselves together". Grace remembered the initiator telling her – in the beginning they were very few (about 15 Grace recalled) – that whenever one of them would "see someone running around", they should inform them about the club and offer them to run together. After time went by the club was growing and more and more people came together, ran together, stretched

---

10   For a more detailed description of the Health Management Information System, see chapter two.

11   The recommended cut-off values by the American Diabetes Association (ADA 2016) are 7,2 mmol/L and 126mg/dL respectively (see chapter one).

together, and "we became somewhat like a family." They organized a coach, who can give some instructions on which exercises are the most profit-yielding.

By the time I met Grace in 2016, the "family" had grown to nearly 250 members. Today the registered club is officially Bo-Health Club. The members of the club are a total mixture of people: young people, older people, female and male, lawyers, engineers, nurses, teachers and "then also these ones really down there. But if you find us together, you cannot tell. The ones who are wealthy, or poor, you would not know, we wear a uniform." Grace was appointed as the general secretary of Bo-Health Club and is "very proud to serve the people". Since it is a limited company, and they do not have support from the government, all the money they need, as for instance to offer free diabetes testing, they have to raise themselves. Part of this money comes from the membership fees each individual has to pay in order to enroll in the club. On payment, an induvial is eligible for a club uniform, including a shirt and some shorts as well as a clubs ID. Grace explained that the fees were so low "because all people in the community should benefit. We do not want to force you to come, and we do not want our fees to chase you away", she said. Subscribing to Bo-Health Club meant to engage in running and stretching activities lead by experienced instructors. But it "is even more than that. It means to do something good for the people", Grace said.

As part of their training, the members of the health club like to participate in different marathons around town as for instance the yearly MTN[12] marathon. Some of the marathons are for a good cause. Grace described:

> "Nowadays the marathons around Kampala are becoming many and we were thinking we also should organize a marathon, as a club. But we did not have the funds. That was last year [2015]. What we did, we went to a stadium and said we want a marathon. They asked 'A marathon for what'? We said 'Just a marathon'. They said that is a good idea. But they also said it would be better to have a cause to run for. Back then we decided to run for the Uganda Heart Foundation because one of the members had some connections to them. The money we raised was little, but we managed to buy some small equipment for them. For testing for pressure. You know the pressure machines. But it was not very successful, because there was actually no money. You know the expectations were so high."

One year later Bo-Health Club wanted to host another marathon, again for a good cause. Because the outcome of the run they had the previous year was not as successful as they had hoped for, they did not want to "think big" for the 2016

---

12 MTN, Mobile Telephone Networks Group, is a South African based telecommunication agency and one of the main providers in Uganda.

marathon. Since they wanted to focus on another health issue, they were pondering about what they could do to help the community? They sat together and brainstormed. To find out what the "community really needed", a small delegation of members of the health club visited some of the health centers around the area to find out what was needed and "to see what is there." Instead of giving money, they tried to find solutions for problems by actively getting involved in changing a situation for the community. "It is an act for the community. We learn to serve in an act of giving without receiving", the director of Bo-Health Club told me.

That is how they became acquainted with Dr. M., the head of one of the health center IIIs close by. Dr. M. was pleased to hear about the intentions and informed the team that there was an urgent need for "diabetes machines because we do not have any."[13] Dr. M. was the one who explained to the team that when people learned they had diabetes, their health had often already deteriorated. That is why he wanted to raise awareness, sensitize and test people so that they get to know their status before complications had already set in. Grace stressed that now Ugandans were often even more scared of getting diabetes than HIV. "Diabetes and pressure can throw you down, HIV can be with you for some time", she said. Dr. M. insisted on the diabetes testing, even when Grace and her team suggested to offer malaria testing instead. Dr. M. said that diabetes was the most important on the agenda, more important than every other disease. Grace explained that

> "diabetes may seem weird to focus on as compared to other diseases like HIV. But it is like this: when I have a headache, I go and buy a painkiller, I do not go for checkup. When I have a stomach ache, I go and buy a painkiller. Even if I have something else, I will go and buy some painkillers, hoping, it will go away on its own. That is a weakness we have. We are not like you people that when I have a cough I need to first check why I am coughing. The reason why people don't go for checkup is that they often ask for this fee that they do not have so they buy a painkiller with the little money instead. We want to change this thinking by offering checkup for the community for free. Our experience is that people get excited when they hear we are testing for diabetes. It is nothing that is usually tested for in the health facilities. Diabetes is also dangerous because it is quiet. That is the problem. HIV is not so quiet. We wanted to see that the quietness at least breaks open and it opens its eyes."

Together with the rest of the team they soon came up with the slogan "Diabetes is preventable", which would also become the theme of the run. They got on with

---

13 It is important to note that glucometers, though sometimes available in health center IIIs, are not necessarily designated for governmental health facilities lower than health center IV, as I have been told by an employee from NMS, the National Medical Stores, who are responsible for the distribution of medical equipment and pharmaceuticals.

their work, started writing proposals and sent them to different companies hoping they would donate some money and sponsor them. "But you know, when you are not yet up there like MTN, bigger companies usually do not want to work with you. They prefer the bigger companies that are already established", she reasoned. Some companies donated money, two others contributed with water for the marathon. A few private people also gave some money, but the outcome was not what they had expected or hoped for.

July the 17th 2016 the big day had come, the day the marathon was taking place. "It was like a big eye opener. The most important thing, it was a run for the community. The town's mayor was the chief runner", Grace recalled. The fee to participate in the run was 10.000 UGX[14]. Since around 500 people participated, deducting all the expenses prior to the run, they had a surplus of around 2,5 Mio. UGX[15]. That was almost double the profit compared to the previous year. They were able to buy two glucometers as well as 1500 testing strips from the money they raised.[16] When they handed over the donations to Dr. M., he decided to "give it back to the community". That is how it came to the 'roadside testing' on that one day when I was actually on my way to health center IV in district X. Having the glucometers enabled them to invite people to come for testing, considering that the next possible place to test was in Kampala or at private facilities. They saw it as their responsibility to help their community, where they had the feeling that the government was failing. Grace explicated:

> "We are a bigger support than the government and that is why we are doing all of this. It [diabetes] is creeping so we have the feeling we need to do something. I am so glad to be part of something that is doing good in the community. God loves people and he is the one who has created all of them. Usually we have the feeling, that the bazungus, the Whites, for them they have a heart of giving. But God also requires us Ugandans to do something. I may not have a lot, but with what I have, what can I do with this little?"

When I visited Dr. M., in his health center two weeks after the outreach, he told me that the two glucometers that were donated to the health center from Bo-Health Club were by no means the first glucometers the health center had seen. In 2014,

---

14 Approximately 2,70 US Dollars.
15 Approximately 684 US Dollars.
16 When talking to the laboratory technician I was told that usually they order 10 tins of glucose strips with each 25 testing strips for two months, making 125 glucose strips for one month for the whole health center. But, as he explained, the first half of tins can get used up on only one day if the patients are many. Therefore 1500 testing strips – which equal the amount of testing strips for a whole year – can be seen as an enormous amount as compared to what governmental facilities have at their disposal.

they received a glucometer from PEPFAR[17], but after the strips got finished, it could no longer be used. A year later, a nearby church donated another glucometer, a different brand with different strips, but the same thing happened: the strips ran out and there was no chance to get new ones. "And after all," he said, "people usually do not come here for testing because they know there is no medicine."

The testing strips were provided for to last for a good amount of time and in case the strips would run out, "there is always a way to get new ones with the help of good people in the club", Grace said. "We are doing this here because not everybody knows that health is important. Basically, we are jumping in for all those ministers who are not doing their job", she said. They have big plans, Dr. M. together with the team of Bo-Health Club: they want to establish a diabetes clinic for the health center with the money they raise with the next marathon. Within the next three to four years, people shall be able to come to a new diabetes clinic for testing: "It is an act for our community, which will be good for all of us. We want to be healthy in our hearts, and want people around us to be healthy too. Whatever is in our capacity we will do."

This section differed from the first section in terms of the initiators of the outreach. A sports club set this outreach in motion intending to do something for the health of the community. In consultation with a medical practitioner, they decided to put their efforts and the money they raised into an outreach that offers free diabetes testing. The doing good from within, was seen to be a substitute and a way to stand in for the people who the Ministry of Health of Uganda seemed to neglect. Yet like the first empirical vignette hinted at and like it will be the case in the last empirical section, here too there was no medication offered for individuals. Outreaches as a means to diagnose diabetes without providing aftercare also has ethical implications. Especially the next part will scrutinize the discrepancy between the will to do good and the effects this doing good may have when people are diagnosed with life-threatening glucose levels, but there is no subsequent care provided.

"The money is totally worth the experience"

The laboratory technicians in seemed very excited, when I arrived there one Tuesday morning. I wondered what was going on, what the reason for the cheerful atmosphere was. A team of doctors from the US was back again to Uganda to screen

---

17 PEPFAR, the "President's Emergency Plan for AIDS Relief", is preoccupied with matters surrounding HIV and AIDS. However, it was not the first time that I an organization got involved in e.g. diabetes. As we have seen in the first sub-chapter in the example of the Family Health Days.

people in a few selected villages of the district, I was told. "Back *again*?", I asked. "Oh yes", someone replied, "twice a year they are coming to Uganda helping us, especially with good technology, and we catch many people. You will be happy, Arlena, they also test for sukali [diabetes]", one of the laboratory technicians told me. In this health facility, they had not been testing for diabetes since months due to the stock out of testing strips – respectively due to the fact that the glucometer they were using was outdated and the strips could no longer be provided by the government. I must admit that I was also happy and infected with the excitement that filled the air of the laboratory, though not really knowing what to expect. One of the health care workers told me "it is a blessing that these people come every year. Especially with the sukali [diabetes] testing. This is something we cannot do here at this hospital at the moment." I would join this team of doctors from the US for a weekend in August 2015 for the first time, and a second time the following year.

It was a sunny morning when I was on my way from Kampala to district X where I would meet and pick up some of the staff from the laboratory who would complement the US outreach team. It was 7.30 a.m. on a Saturday morning, when I reached the Health Center from where we would start out to the first village on a one-hour drive. Taking a slope to the left off the main road, along an enormous bumpy mud road, up a hill (though I floored the accelerator, the car could not drive faster than about 20 km/h, also because the car was packed with people and equipment), past a few trading centers, where people were selling vegetables and fruit. Fewer and fewer people were walking along the roadside, the further we left the health center behind. I remember how stunned I was when we arrived at the primary school of this village, where the screening was to be held. Masses of people had come to be tested for the different diseases. Later we would find out that it was a total of about 700 people who had come for testing only on this one day. A bodaboda driver was driving past the school compound with a megaphone, blazing abroad, while Charly, one of the laboratory technicians, was translating what the man was calling: "Come and test. Come for check-up. You should not miss this chance, doctors have come from abroad. They are bazungus [travelers from abroad], come and test."

It transpired that the alleged team of doctors from the US was by no means the like. Instead the team involved a Professor for biochemistry, Professor Jim, followed by his wife and a small group of eight undergraduate students between the age of 19 and 24. The Professor and his wife were themselves Ugandans, but living and working in the US since the end of the 1980s. He told me that he of course knew very well where the shortcomings were within Uganda's health care system, which is why he has been coming back to his home country twice a year to visit some of the villages in district X and offer screening for a range of diseases: hypertension, HIV, malaria and diabetes. Medical counseling and the provision of some medication like antimalarial, painkillers, deworming tablets and vitamins was offered as well, all free of charge. Drugs for diabetes were, however, not offered.

What had initially started out as an exchange program between students of microbiology, biochemistry and laboratory science who would come from the US to learn together with students from Uganda and vice versa, soon became an integral part of his teaching efforts since nearly 15 years. Though different students accompanied him every time he traveled to Uganda, his vision stayed the same, he wanted to bring back some of the knowledge gained from the laboratory in the US to his mother country and teach the students "who do not really know what is happening deep in the villages". He had the permission from the municipality to conduct the outreaches as "we could not simply come here and test the people without anybody knowing", he explained. Later on, I spoke to one of the medical directors of the municipality, who told me that the district was profiting from the project. It would always bring some donor equipment such as a scale or some glucometers that the Professor would leave with them.

In the US, Professor Jim was conducting research on metabolic diseases, non-communicable diseases and nutrition-related diseases using animal models to understand the complex mechanisms of nutrient-genetic interaction and to see which foods were beneficial when managing, delaying or preventing non-communicable diseases. Diabetes was the disease, which interested him most and it were especially countries like Uganda, he reasoned, where early prevention and detection were crucial for it would take people long until they sought medical care. That is why he decided to go into the communities as "most of the problems can be found there [and because] resources are low and diagnosing is poor". Since 2002, however, when Professor Jim had left his old university to continue his career at another, he was still bringing students from the US twice a year (around January and again around July) but they were studying different subjects such as Gender Studies or Zoology, thus not medicine-related. One reason why the students came all the way from the US to Uganda for two weeks, was that they received a certificate for attending the trip to Uganda. A certificate in 'Global Health' and additionally two credit points to complete their transcript of records for their undergraduate studies. For all of them it was the first time in Uganda, even the first time on the African continent and for some it was the first time far away from home. Yet talking to students revealed that they saw their trip as an adventure, "perhaps the once in a lifetime chance to come to Africa", one of them said. Though, as another student added, "it was very sad to see all the poverty and see the people suffering from diseases like HIV" and that "the only thing keeping me sane, is that they are getting help and that's amazing."

The trip came with costs. One of the students told me she had paid around 2000 US Dollars for the flight plus 2800 US Dollars for the two weeks' trip, which included accommodation[18], food, a safari to Murchison Falls[19], as well as the three-day outreach-weekend to the villages where "we help the village people". "But", she explained, "the money is totally worth the experience because we get to do a lot of things we are not allowed to do in the US. Technically we are not even allowed to be doing what we are doing", she confessed, with a sly smile. It was not only the first time in Uganda for the students, but it was the first time they would draw blood and test human beings for life threatening diseases like HIV, malaria and diabetes – without previous training on how to use the technology[20].

The testing started at around 8.30 a.m. The different testing stations had been prepared beforehand. School desks had been carried outside the classrooms onto the schoolyard and everything was arranged in a way so that each disease had its own space on the compound and the people could approach the stations one after the other. All the medical equipment[21] was brought along by Professor Jim from the US, except the HIV and malaria testing kits, which had been ordered and bought at a pharmacy in Kampala. The glucometers the Professor had brought were brand new and "up-to-date", as he told me. One strip alone was worth between two and three dollars, an "enormous amount of money for the village people here", he said. The machines were donations from his friends who were working as medical doctors in hospitals or had a private practice in the US. Gym bags filled with boxes of glucometers and extra packages of glucose testing strips, medical devices that would be taken back to the US after they had fulfilled their purpose of testing people. For "accountability reasons" as the Professor explained. How many health facilities in the district could be catered for with these machines? Donated technology that was so valuable in many places of the country.

Before the people could be tested, each of them had to be registered at the registration station: name, age, sex and village were noted down by one of the American students. The next station took care of taking the vitals, which included measuring the blood pressure and taking the pulse. Station three was for HIV testing, station four for malaria testing and station five for diabetes testing. Then there

---

18 Later on, I was told that the Professor had built a large house in the district, where he could accommodate all the students he brought to Uganda twice a year and he owned a bus, which would transport them from place to place with a driver.
19 Murchison Falls is one of the National Parks in Uganda and one of the places to go for safari.
20 Not knowing how to use the technology properly was accompanied with some problems. For example, because the students did not know and were not instructed how to properly draw blood, some of the people had to be pricked several times, a painful and unnecessary act. Another incident was that one of the students unintentionally pricked herself with a needle after she had used it to test a person for diabetes. She feared having contracted an infectious disease. I heard the wife of Professor Jim whispering "I told you these kids shouldn't be dealing with needles."
21 A scale to take the weight; a measuring tape for measuring the height; glucometers to measure the blood glucose; pens to write and sheets of paper to document; needles for pricking etc.

were two additional stations, one headed by an optometrist for eye exams and the other by a dentist assistant for an inspection of the teeth. Finally, the mobile dispensary where common drugs like painkillers, antimalarial, antibiotics and vitamins could be dispensed, rounded up the offered services of the two-day outreach program. Individuals could decide freely which station they wanted to approach and whether they wanted to be tested for all the diseases available only wanted for certain diseases. Children were generally not screened for hypertension (blood pressure) or diabetes. The stations where, as the students put it "real testing" or the "real stuff" was taking place, was more attractive for them compared to weighing people or measuring the height, which they described as "rather boring." One student preened herself on her experiences she had collected in a retirement home in the US, where she had done an internship. "I am already quite experienced in taking care of people, I was allowed to take the temperature and measure the blood pressure during my internship", she told me proudly.

The stations of HIV and malaria testing were supported by each two laboratory technicians. They had brought the documentation books in which every malaria and HIV test (no matter whether positive or negative) was noted down. Not so for diabetes. In fact, as compared to Health Centers Y and Z where NCD registration books are used, the Ministry of Health of Uganda has generally not yet provided a means for documentation for health centers who are not part of the project of the Medical Research Council. What was then happening with the data generated for diabetes as well as hypertension if there was no formal way to capture it and hand it over to the districts data manager? When I asked the districts data manager some weeks after the outreach, he had not yet received any data on diabetes (or hypertension).

As a matter of course, I decided to stay at the diabetes station, which was installed next to a tree. For the individuals to be able to identify it as the diabetes station, a sheet of paper with "Awakebererwa sukali" ('blood sugar testing point') written on it had been pinned to the tree. Due to the high influx of people coming to the station, one of the students was engaged in noting down the testing results on the individual's registration sheet as well as on a separate sheet, which documented all the people who had visited the station. Glucose levels above 120 mg/dL were additionally underlined on a separate sheet so that Professor Jim could later on easily identify the cases with elevated glucose levels. Usually individuals were only tested when they were above 35. However, since it was still early in the morning and there were many testing strips available, the Professor decided to test everybody who wanted to be tested for diabetes who was 18 years and above. Also, because "we should capture as many as possible to get a big picture", he said.

The testing itself followed a similar procedure I had observed so many times before. In order to put the glucometer to use, there is no necessity of having a fully equipped laboratory. The glucometer can work anywhere and it can allegedly be used by anybody to test anybody: you take a strip from the small tin, insert the strip into the strip slot of the glucometer. A beep confirms that the strip has been inserted correctly. Then another beep followed by a symbol resembling a drop of blood on the screen of the machine asks the user to apply a drop of blood onto the strip. It then sucks up the blood from the fingertip. When enough blood is applied, the machine will beep again to confirm that there has been enough blood applied. Then the countdown of six seconds starts: 6, 5, 4, 3, 2, 1, until a number appears on the screen of the device: the glucose level of the tested person. Professor Jim was always very eager to be the first to see the individuals with "the high numbers." After all, identifying individuals with diabetes was the reason for his coming, it was what he was interested in. That is why he stood or sat close to the diabetes station most of the times to be there, whenever an individual would have a glucose level above 120 mg/dL. I remember him literally tearing the paper out of the student's hand who was documenting, when a person was obviously older than 35 or overweight. "How much is she?", "What is the level?", "Is he ok?", were questions he frequently asked when the two indicators age and weight matched. When the level was below 120 mg/dL, he almost sounded surprised saying "oh, only so little?", as if he had been certain the person must be having diabetes; as if he could see diabetes in the person's eyes; almost, as if he could not believe the glucometer was giving the right result. Though a certain age and weight increase the probability of diabetes, as they are two of the risk factors, it does not automatically mean a person will have diabetes.

What was done with and for the individuals who did have elevated glucose levels? I remember two incidences very well. It was one of the first people coming to the station that day. On first sight, I thought it was a child. He handed over his registration sheet to one of the students, while the other prepared herself to test him. It turned out he was a 40-year-old man, 24 kg light[22]. The student who was testing took one of his fingers, pricked him, applied the drop of blood onto the glucose strip and then, six seconds later, the device indicated '>600 mg/dL'. The device gave instructions to repeat the test. Again: above 600 mg/dL. The glucometer screen displayed the words "Over 600 mg/dL Again. Follow Medical Advice Immediately".

Glucometers are usually not able to measure a glucose level beyond 600 mg/dL. Everyone was shocked. Professor Jim did not hesitate to gently take the man's arm, pull him aside a bit and say "olina sukali", meaning "you have diabetes" in Luganda. I remember very well that the man was repeating the words "ndi bulungi", translatable with "but I am ok". This small device indicated a number that in turn indicated a disease and in turn gave reason to diagnose diabetes, a life-changing moment on this day for this man who actually did not feel sick.

---

[22] One of the side effects of an uncontrolled glucose level over a long period is the loss of weight, also see chapter one.

The second instance of an overly high blood sugar level was an 18-year-old female. One of the two students at the station noted down her name, the other was putting on a fresh pair of blue rubber gloves. After the young lady was tested, the glucometer indicated a blood sugar level of 560 mg/dL the first time. She was tested again to double-check. This time the glucometer could not display the result (it must have exceeded the 600 by far) but only indicated 'HI'[23], an abbreviation for high blood glucose level. As did the result of the glucose test of the man in the example before, this result was worrying. In fact, such a high glucose level requires immediate medical attention and action. But the only thing that could be done at that moment in this location was to take her to the medical clinical officer, who was responsible to give advice and initiate care in form of giving medicine, it was available at this time in this place. It turned out that the young woman was aware that she had diabetes, therefore the diagnosis did not come as a surprise. She explained that she had stopped taking her medication three months ago. The health center nearby the village, a health center II, did not have the means to take care of individuals with diabetes. They could not test at that health center II, nor did they have the medication needed to treat this disease. She told us that she would have to travel far to a bigger health center, which was costly. Later in the evening, the watch hand had already passed 7 p.m., darkness had covered the country, and we were sitting in the car on our way back home, tired from the day, filled with impressions and happenings, George said: "I cannot believe there were two people today who almost died on the spot with such high glucose levels." What about the laboratory technicians who were supporting the outreach team of the Professor? One of them later told me, they received a small allowance. Money, many of them urgently needed, considering the fact that most of them were waiting for their salaries for months already. But there was another thing some of them received: a glucometer and each ten strips. The other glucometers would travel back to the US, they had fulfilled their temporary purpose.

This last empirical vignette brought us to the compound of a village school. Testing for different diseases was offered by a team of Americans who had come to do good, especially by offering testing for diabetes. This outreach, compared to the other two, was a lot bigger in scope. What was lacking or not functioning in the first example of this chapter, could be found in abundance especially in this last example: glucometers. Yet, we also were able to see that twice individuals had such high glucose levels that immediate medical action would have needed to follow. This was, however, not possible due to the locality of the village, the next health

---

23 The manual of the glucometer explains that if a test result is displayed as HI [high] or LO [low] immediate medical attention is required by a doctor. This also shows that the testing result displayed by one and the same glucometer may vary within just a few minutes, though the test is performed allegedly in the same way with the same device.

center that could treat diabetes far away. We have met a team whose actions may critically questioned. Was the good they intended to do really good? For whom were they good? Testing for diabetes always involves the danger that glucose levels are in fact health or even life threatening and require actions taken to counteract high glucose levels. We will have the chance to discuss the findings of these three empirical sections in the final part of this chapter.

Desired tests, undesired outcomes?

This chapter has taken us to three different settings where, next to screening other diseases, diabetes testing was offered. Diabetes has found its way into the minds of people and the awareness of this condition seems to rise. That the testing for "sukali" (diabetes) attracted and excited so many people as "a crowd puller" reflects this trend. Though the three examples of outreaches presented in this chapter diverge in scope, their initial intentions, the locality of testing, the resources available etc., they are tied together by their engagement in screening for diabetes against the backdrop of diabetes being a silent disease, that has to be revealed before disturbing symptoms show themselves when the disease is already in a progressed state. It is testing by chance rather than testing as a result of a tangible indication. All three outreaches offered testing under the premise of screening as a preventive rather than a curative measure. What followed after the testing was – in case an individual had a high glucose level – offering advice, but not initiating care in form of a (pharmaceutical) therapy. The outreaches we have seen here are bound to a certain locality, where testing occurs in a certain place while medications in the case of a diagnosis of diabetes, respectively the assumption of an existing diabetes, have to be given in another.

The first example has taken us to a pharmacy in a trading center close to the health center IV in district X. This outreach was the remnant of a larger project, the "Family Health Days", which were carried out in the district previously as part of a cooperation between UNICEF and the Ministry of Health of Uganda in places of worship, such as churches. The Family Health Days, which targeted children in the first place, were used as a platform, to offer screening for a disease where numerical evidence was still lacking and the need was seen to engage in activities that work on this disease by the Ministry of Health of Uganda. The setting, churches and places of worship, were perceived to have a positive influence on the acceptance and accessibility within the community. A lot less effort was involved as well as the barrier lowered for those, who feared governmental services where "they get rude and unfriendly." The second example presented in this chapter brought us to a roadside testing site by coincidence; I was actually on my way to the health center in district X, when the happenings on the roadside drew my attention. The members of a sports club, the Bo-Health Club, decided to host a marathon for a "good cause". Together with a medical doctor from a nearby health center they focused their testing efforts on diabetes as the doctor certified that this was the disease for which there was the biggest need. According to Grace, one of the members of the health club, it was an act of giving out of charity and a standing in for what the ministry of health was perceived of failing to offer: testing for diabetes. In the third example finally, we found ourselves in a village school of district X, where a team together with a few health care workers from a health center IV offered comprehensive screening for malaria, HIV, hypertension[24] and especially for diabetes. The abundance of glucometers and testing strips reflected the personal efforts and research interests of Professor Jim. A Ugandan himself living in the US, he wanted to bring back knowledge to his home country, knowingly that prevention and detection of disease are essential especially in chronic diseases like diabetes, a disease that takes people long until they sought medical care.

I have suggested to view medical outreaches in terms of taking the chance of securing medical equipment, funds and social networks when the opportunity opens up against the backdrop of a disease, which has largely been neglected by the local government and international organization. Outreaches as a humanitarian endeavor draw their justification exactly from the tension between temporarily increasing the access to diagnostic and treatment technologies on the one hand. On the other hand, it is assumed that this will a have positive effect for an individual and a health care system when a disease is grabbed in its beginnings and is made visible. The quote by writer and philosopher Albert Camus (1955) stated in the introduction of this chapter "Seeking what is true is not seeking what is desirable", raises an important issue, which allows us to reflect upon medical outreaches with a critical gaze: is screening for disease an undertaking, which is desirable? There is no straightforward answer. Screening tests seek to create evidence of disease in populations and/or individuals, where a disease has not been anticipated. Or, it has been anticipated, but the technological means have been missing. Grounded on the assumption that not only the individual will profit from the early discovery of the disease in a state where harmful side effects are still preventable and disease treatable; the whole health care system will profit when disease is uncovered early and therapeutic measures are still less expensive (Jutel 2011; Armstrong 1995; Nelkin and Tancredi 1989, 1994).

Research on medical outreaches is limited (exemptions are e.g. Eliasoph 2011; Hilton and McKay 2011). While screening for disease has found its way into medical

---

24 Interestingly in all three outreaches offered screening for malaria and HIV next to diabetes testing. This on the one hand can be seen as the attempt to cover as many potential diseases as possible. It can, however, also be read in terms of justifying diabetes screening exactly because screening for malaria and HIV were also offered.

practice, there is an ongoing debate about whether the detriments of medical outreaches outweigh the benefits or vice versa. What resonates with screening latently is the assumption, that screening is something that is desired by the individuals or populations who receive the screening. Quotes from individuals I have met such as "we are doing good", or "it is an act of giving" assert this. As Jutel describes "on the surface, it would hardly seem problematic to detect what might be silent for now but disease later" (Jutel 2011: 128), but there might be effects of such undertakings, including a longer phase of morbidity especially in chronic diseases like diabetes, which cannot be assessed beforehand. It has also been added for consideration that a potential rivalry or competition between ordinary health care services and screening services may arise (Jutel 2011; Black 2000). As it presented itself during the outreaches, especially by the Bo-Health Club was that the outreach was perceived not as competitive to the governmental services available, but as complementary for lacking infrastructures for chronic diseases. Following Mol (2002) diseases – and here I subjoin the *diagnosis* of diseases – are performed through practices and routines that are coordinated and cohered by rules and guidelines. Yet if these rules or guidelines, are missing, there is space for improvisation. Members of a health club may become the main actors when planning a roadside screening for diabetes and students from the US who study Gender Studies back home might come and test for diabetes (and other diseases) without any prior medical experience.

As stated before, screening generally aims at detecting disease at an early stage and initiate care timely. The fact that screening, or medical outreaches as they are usually called in Uganda, are offered outside the average health care services on the roadside, outside a church or on the compound of a primary school is accompanied by a significant aspect: the accessibility and reachability to diagnostics is increased and individuals who would not have had access to testing, are now easier reached. The significance is reinforced in the case of diabetes, where testing and care is often limited to but not necessarily available at higher health facilities. Therefore, outreaches might spawn an incongruity between outreaches as a valuable tool by bringing the clinic to underserved settings contrasted by the fact that screening during outreach programs might pose a greater burden on the health care system which has to handle an increased number of patients yielded by these practices. There is an ambivalence between uncovering disease as a good deed and uncovering diseases against the backdrop of a lack of services. Like Dr. M. said, "people usually do not come here for testing because they know there is no medicine."

The alleged simplicity of point-of-care devices such as the glucometer (which can also easily be used by non-medical personnel) used for instance for diabetes testing – small drop of blood, wait for the result and then it will be displayed on the screen of the glucometer – may overshadow and obscure the fact that a human being's life is at stake. Lupton states that "while patients subscribe to the notion that technological investigation of symptoms provides an objective diagnosis, the medical discourse obscures the social forces shaping the test result" (Lupton 2001: 154). The result of a preventive screening test may turn out positive and the devastating outcomes of a positive test have to be dealt with by an individual as well as the ones diagnosing (ibid.). Misperformance as well as unthoughtful use of technology might outweigh the benefits and have far reaching implications (see also Manderson et al. 2016). The motivation of an individual to seek care, like a disturbing symptom, is missing in screening. Yet it functions as a way "to delete the possibility of disease", as one of the individuals stated. When such a test turns out "negative", meaning the glucose levels are in the range, it will leave a person with a good feeling.

This presumptive testing might, as was the case in one of the individuals with a high glucose level cause more of a shocking moment followed by anxiety as compared to when an individual comes to a health center seeking for a diagnosis and hoping to find an answer to ones' pains. What about the individuals that came for the free testing, either not expecting to be sick, like it was the case for the 40-year-old man described above, or who already knew they had diabetes like it was the case for the young woman, who then were told they had "sukali". In fact, there was nothing more the outreach team could offer than the testing. Testing to uncover disease may come with anxiety. One individual even decided not to be tested out of fear diabetes might be revealed. Black (2000) too raises concerns about the detection of a disease, which would have "gone to the grave with the patient (while not being the cause of death), [resulting] in anxiety" (Black 2000, in Jutel 2001: 128).

DeCamp defines the goal of global short-term outreaches as the provision of "tangible medical benefits to individuals in the community" (DeCamp 2007: 21), whereby who benefits and how a community benefits may be critically questioned. This is why medical outreaches as we have seen in the third example raises ethical questions. Under the guise of "doing good", or "we help the village people" the outreach served as a playground, a living laboratory (Tilley 2011) for students who, compared to the ethical limitations of medical testing in their home country, were allowed to test people. Offering services for individuals who would otherwise not have known of their disease, screening for disease, while practiced with great endeavor, might not always be carried out with the individual knowing. Though there was medicine for malaria, some painkillers and nutrients available at the mobile pharmacy, medicine to treat diabetes was missing in the pharmacy. Patients who were told they had diabetes, were required to go to the next health center to fetch medicines from there, though the closest one, a health center II, too could not offer the care or testing needed. People were diagnosed against the backdrop of stock outs of medicine as well as a lacking glucose measurement device in the district's main health center IV. People were diagnosed, knowingly, that the necessary infrastructures were not in place to be able to handle the disease.

This chapter did not focus on the experience of a diagnosis itself, but aimed to picture the implementation of screening practices in diverse settings by exploring the social and structural contexts to which they were applied. Hereby it is important to consider that the implementing parties and actors involved, who carried out the screening, had their own agendas, which disease(s) to screen, where, and how, influenced by individual interests, political decisions as well as structural preconditions: offering the testing for diabetes and hypertension as a crowd puller so that parents brought their children for vaccination and provision of vitamins; as an act of giving without receiving and stepping in for a government that is perceived to fail in delivering sufficient services for diabetes; or offering diabetes testing for personal research interests while at the same time providing students a platform on which they can collect experiences, which they could not get in their home country. What connects all of these screening efforts was the ambition to uncover disease before it has manifested itself and – to repeat the quote of a health worker – "to bring the clinic to the villages". As DeCamp offers for consideration, testing, or technology in general, cannot be seen as a panacea for inequalities in global health and "problems addressed in short-term medical outreach are only symptoms of broader inequalities in health that require more radical solutions at the national and international level" (DeCamp 2007: 22).

While screening may be seen as an alternative or complementary way of diagnosing disease where the services are insufficient or lacking in a health care system, good intentions do not necessarily lead to beneficiary outcomes for the individuals who are tested. Screening, which holds the chance of diagnosing disease, may transform a former healthy body into a body with disease. Especially a disease like diabetes requires the immediate referral to ongoing services in case disease is suspected, and herewith the possibility of initiating treatment and continuous care after a diagnosis has been made. To repeat the words of Dr. K.: "It is not only about screening but also about the capacity of the health care system to deliver the required service. You wonder if it is good to know and die or you do not know and die? I don't know. Unless you deliver that service, it is not enough to just screen.

Concluding Remarks

Despite the increasing awareness and advances knowledge- and technological wise, the incidence and prevalence of diabetes continues to be on the rise worldwide. A large number of people living with diabetes hereby remains undiagnosed or poorly treated (Chatterjee et al. 2017: 2239). We have reached the final part of this book. However, we still cannot be sure which particular circumstances caused the specific death of George, whose story I retold in the introduction. Maybe the lack of equipment to test his blood sugar levels, or perhaps insufficient knowledge to interpret his symptoms appropriately. Nevertheless, I took this fatal incident as a starting point to draw an in-depth picture of the context, the conditions and circumstances under which he died, and the complexities in which individuals like George, their caregivers and technologies like the glucometer, are entangled in Ugandan diabetes care. The story of George and all the other individuals we met throughout this book might be local stories. Yet they have proven to be no less global. These (hi)stories are, or ought to be, a global matter. Diabetes is no longer merely a concern of the minority world as was long perceived. In fact, it has to find its way into the minds of scholars, politicians and activists. Likewise, in the majority *and* the minority world. Diabetes and other chronic diseases are a 'new' global threat and burden of the 21st century. Yet countries in the majority world suffer disproportionally, struggling to provide even the most basic equipment and care.

This book has focused on the glucometer as a medical device and actor in the field of global health. It has set out with the initial question of what a technology like this can render visible in the contested and entangled field of global health politics. Visibility of a disease is key to health systems. Diagnosing and treatment requires visibility. Visibility enables the identification of needs, and is thus an inherently political issue. Documenting the glucometer as it is used by different actors in various application sites showed that applying this device is both, an achievement as well as it is an ambiguous enterprise. What the device reveals or what remains hidden depends on the setting to which it is applied as well as on the actors who engage in its use. In this sense, the study is a medical anthropological autopsy, identifying layers of global context, actors, their relations and knowledges, whose practices and effects on health outcomes evolve, and can only be understood empirically. The following remarks conclude this book and bring the central findings together. In three sub-sections, I scrutinize the core aspects that have become apparent in the empirical chapters. Finally, we will turn our gaze forwards to discuss what these findings might mean within the struggle for visibility and the politics of diabetes diagnostics in Uganda and beyond.

Contesting the global health agenda

Global health is not a straightforward and unproblematic approach towards the health and the wellbeing of the global public. Actions within the field of global health should be critically assessed concerning the moral and ideological implications of its actors. For example, the prioritization of infectious diseases occurs at the expense of chronic diseases – both in terms of medical interventions taking place as well as the financial aid that is provided. I have shown that the current way the global health agenda is constituted has consequences for improving the health and care of diabetes. In the case of chronic diseases, we may therefore particularly doubt its global reach. To put it frankly: How 'global' is global health really? Why are much of the urgently required efforts taken locally? In fact, compared to diseases, which are geographically bound to certain areas such as malaria or Ebola, diabetes is more global than these diseases are and perhaps ever will be. Nevertheless, global action characterizes disease interventions for tropical infectious diseases such as Ebola or malaria. Diabetes on the other hand is not attached to a geographic area, but is prevalent in every country across the globe. It is in the truest sense of the word 'global' and yet still lacks global attention and action plans.

Part of the problem of why diabetes is struggling for visibility in Uganda and beyond is that we live in a world, where numbers are often valorized more than anything else and policies are expected to be evidence-based. The strive for numerical evidence is omnipresent, informing and guiding essential decisions in diverse fields – thus also in global health. Numbers indeed have convincing power, and they are indispensable in many aspects of global health. This book has however demonstrated that there is also the need to understand and appreciate the way in which these numbers are fabricated and how they are following unequal premises across the globe. I have argued that diabetes and other chronic conditions in Uganda are caught in a vortex of suspense. They find themselves within the discrepancy of stagnant policies and the fight for recognition as a result of restricted access to diagnostic tools and a lack of numerical evidence, which ultimately result in scarce (global) financial aid and unevenly distributed visibility of diabetes. The conditions under which numerical evidence can be generated is accordingly not only a matter of good will, or the outcome of best medical practice, it is dependent on (health) infrastructures. One essential way to contribute to the visibility of disease is surely its diagnosis, or testing for it respectively. This is the reason why I located the glucometer as the main actor of this book: it contributes, facilitates or exacerbates the visibility of diabetes in one way or the other. The way data is generated or not generated, or why countries struggle to generate this data altogether cannot be answered by looking at numbers alone. It requires to attend to the circumstances, to which technologies like the glucometer are applied.

Trajectories of a fluid technology

The travel of biomedical technologies on a global scale has increased the availability of medical devices in the majority world. While the diagnostic possibilities subsequently grow, implementing a technology may solve problems, while creating new ones at the same time. Not to mention that not all devices that seemingly travel under the guise of being a diagnostic device are in fact made for diagnosis. Chapter four has dealt with the question what happens when a global health technology like the glucometer travels to a country distinct in its sociotechnical context from the country it originated from. The main task of medical technologies is to assist in care practices or make them possible in the first place. Hereby they hold a promise and raise expectations that they actually *can* improve a condition, which would not possible without these technologies (Nelkin and Tancredi 1994).

By highlighting different aspects surrounding the practicalities and the intended use of the glucometer as stated in glucometer user manuals, I have shown that the use of the glucometer is not an act of mere technology transfer. Structural circumstances may complicate the implementation of the device as we have also seen in other parts of this book (chapter four to six). The de-contextualized promise the glucometer held initially – to measure glucose levels and diagnose diabetes – turned into a dilemma of actually having a technology and being unable to use it properly. Without batteries, glucose strips and the knowledge of how to translate the result literally and analytically, the device is deprived of its functions and will be nothing more than a technology. It cannot be used at all or not to its full extent. It is against this backdrop that translations of the device will take place. Translations in this case take on the character of justifications. Justifying and making sense of the use of the glucometer in a way that it serves as many individuals as possible. The device then transforms, or is transformed, into a device that diagnoses individuals, when it initially has not been meant for diagnosing. It is then also possible to use the device for testing several people, though it is meant to be used by only one person. I suggested that in order to account for the varying translations of the device, aspects of care have to be considered. How actors are able to use the device, how they struggle to keep using it or in fact are unable to use the glucometer, is connected to the translations of the device and influences the way care is provided. Using the glucometer is not only a matter of access, but it involves creative ways to adapt the technology to the given circumstances and with this enabling care practices and keeping them going.

That the glucometer, however, is often the only technology to diagnose diabetes, increases the complexity of the problem. Therefore, chapter five examined the diagnosis of diabetes in different settings. One of the first responses to disease is diagnosis. Ideally, medical uncertainty is replaced by the certainty of what has caused the troubling symptoms and condition. Treatment will be initiated and after some time of convalescence, an individual will be cured. This is not the case for diabetes. Diabetes can be managed, but not cured. Symptoms can be alleviated, but they will remain part of the lifeworlds of the affected individuals. Sorting things out by identifying and categorizing symptoms, and providing an individual with a suitable disease is the main outcome of the medical encounter between an individual seeking care and a health professional providing it (Smith-Morris 2016). Unlike diseases where the interpretation of symptoms may justify a suspected diagnosis and treatment, the diagnosis and testing for diabetes emerges from an interplay between the knowledge of the disease, in terms of its clinical manifestations, and the availability and application of technology. Only if these components come together, a diagnosis can be established. If either the knowledge or the device is lacking, so it seems, a diagnosis is impossible. But there was more to it than the interplay between technology and knowledge that enabled the diagnosis of diabetes.

I have demonstrated that in the quest for a diagnosis it does not matter whether an individual has the means to access private health care or is reliant on governmental health services. Against the neoliberal assumption that more money increases the choices an individual can make and likewise enhances the probability of being diagnosed with diabetes in an earlier stage, I have argued that receiving a diagnosis in Uganda follows a logic of chance. It is less a matter of choice or money, than a matter of chance, whether an individual receives a diagnosis. The chance of meeting the right person, being in the right place at the right time, or the chance of being at a hospital where knowledge and technology coincide. It is especially the post-diagnosis phase, where economic investments can facilitate and expand an individual's option to take care of her- or himself in the new life with a chronic disease. Circumventing long waiting hours and tiring visits in governmental health facilities in Uganda, where medication and equipment is scarce is one possibility; purchasing a private glucometer and engage in self-monitoring practices would be another.

The glucometer took on a different role when used by individuals as part of self-monitoring practices, which was the focus of chapter six. Here the glucometer functioned not only as a device to test diabetes and assess too high, too low, or average glucose levels. But it contributed to the visibility of the disease on a very personal level. I have suggested that self-monitoring and the numbers arising thereof cannot be detached from the glucometer. In this sense, the device is not less powerful when it is used by an individual with diabetes compared to medical professionals who engage in its use. The dual and ambivalent character of the device – limiting uncertainty and gaining more predictability about the disease while at the same time creating uncertainty through its maintenance and access – is inherent to the experience of testing and self-monitoring of diabetes in Uganda. Though it has been critically questioned, whether self-monitoring has benefits for the treatment outcomes, the findings of chapter six suggest that self-monitoring is a means to keep up hope and gain a feeling of safety. Being able to self-monitor was a way to replace uncertainty, and gain a feeling of self-reliance and self-efficacy. Numbers might suggest an objective and neutral result, individuals nevertheless attribute specific emotions to specific numbers. Good numbers encouraged good feelings, bad numbers created fear and anxiety. Using the glucometer as part of self-monitoring and the adding of personal value to the numbers it produced a way of coping and mending shattered lives that these diagnoses often caused.

Next to the use of the glucometer for diagnostic and self-monitoring practices, chapter seven has described alternative testing sites outside of a hospital setting. Here the glucometer was applied in the frame of medical outreaches. The logic of chance here takes on another dimension in a health care system, where guidelines and policies of how to deal with diabetes as well as large-scale interventions are lacking. A setting, where a lack of numbers in form of epidemiological evidence may be seen as the justification to engage in practices and define them as complementing or supporting the health care system and 'doing good'. Doing good in the realm of medical outreaches arises from the perception that it is beneficial to offer services for a disease and apply a technology that is otherwise scarce or not available at all. Yet in contradiction of its original intention, by giving access to glucometer in the context of medical outreaches, actors might not strengthen but impair a health care system. Diagnosing more people with diabetes against the backdrop of restricted capacities for caring for those who are already diagnosed exacerbates the problem.

Further I demonstrated that such outreaches might not necessarily benefit the people, but rather the actors who believe they are doing good. Getting access to a 'living laboratory' (Tilley 2011) and being able to gain 'exotic' experience or to do "what would not be allowed at home", might be good for ones' résumé. Nonetheless it raises ethical questions about how much testing should be done, by whom and where? Is it enough to offer testing without having the expertise, just because you can? Is it ethical to test humans, without the expertise or the capacities to take care of them in case a test turns out positive? Glucometers in the hands of more people, will not necessarily lead to more or do more 'good'. The increasing availability of glucometers demands sustainable responses. It demands responsible and proper handling of the device as well as the individuals who are tested, which Uganda's health care system is not yet fully prepared to deliver. The alleged simplicity of the test obfuscates the far-reaching implications and consequences testing for diabetes in fact has.

Re-visiting (in)visibility

Taken together, the book has shown that bringing a glucometer to Uganda is not a mere act of technology transfer and implementation. It is a technology that plays an active part and thus needs to be actively adapted and translated. It is the act of translating the glucometer that helps to make life and care practices easier and keeps diabetes care going. Without a translation of the device, care for diabetes would not or only hardly be possible. The glucometer in a setting like Uganda promises easy and quick testing for diabetes, while at the same time being the only possibility for testing and diagnosing and especially for making diabetes visible in Uganda's health care system and beyond. On the other hand, testing and diagnosing alone are not enough in the case of diabetes. The possibility of testing is entangled with the impossibility to meet the needs of an increase number of individuals with diabetes. A positive diabetes test is the beginning of a life in which numbers and continuous testing are indispensable for the affected individuals to stay alive. The increased number of people suffering from diabetes, calls for an adaptation of health-care systems in the majority world, which are often not well prepared to deal with the high burden of these conditions economically, politically, technologically and knowledge wise. Without testing, there will be no diabetes, or rather no scientifically confirmed case of diabetes, not on paper and not in any records. But without the visibility, knowledge and therefore awareness of the disease, it will not take on the urgency it requires to stand up to the regimes of global health.

How can we proceed from here? One approach that has been suggested is to reorganize and reframe chronic diseases not only as non-communicable diseases, but as diseases that struggle for visibility in the majority world. One of the main differences between infectious and chronic diseases is that chronic diseases seem less threatening. They do not have to be kept at bay, because they might transcend national borders like viruses. As Allen and Feigl (2017) have recently suggested, a renaming of non-communicable diseases is necessary to highlight the urgency these diseases entail. Actions on non-communicable diseases, they argue, may be "hampered by the inadequacy of their label" and have proposed to term NCDs as "socially transmitted conditions (STCs), [which] stresses the anthropogenic and socially contagious nature of the diseases [driven by] urbanization, industrialization, and poverty, the availability of tobacco, alcohol, and processed foods, and physical inactivity" (ibid.: e645). This might be a first step, especially considering that the regimes of global health require a more urgent and imperative language that can be subsumed under the terms of emergency or humanitarian crisis. But will a renaming of non-communicable diseases help to initiate more (global and local) action and generate more funding? Perhaps Allen and Feigl are right when they say that there is little to lose "by abandoning a term that does not resonate with the evidence or the general public" (ibid.). However, a renaming of non-communicable diseases into 'socially transmitted conditions' might in fact only be a way to pour old wine into new bottles and it does not grapple with the infrastructural dimension behind the problem. And who is it really, who still needs to be convinced of the threat chronic diseases pose?

A priority within global health actions is the creation of innovative point-of-care devices that enable diagnostics even in parts of the world with weak laboratory infrastructures. As Moran-Thomas (2017) states "glucose meters stand out as a boundary case example of technological design that has not been transformed", even though they serve for a lot more than for diagnostic purposes of diabetes. The diagnosis of diabetes is just the beginning of a life with a disease, which requires treatment as well as close-meshed and continuous monitoring, if they want to follow best practice recommendations from the medical field. Why, after all, have inexpensive diagnostic devices been manufactured for other diseases but not for diabetes (Moran-Thomas 2017)?

Indeed, historically the glucometer has been designed for countries in the minority world, but it continues to be produced and further developed for these markets. The glucometer has what Benjamin (2015) termed a "discriminatory design". It is a technology with "foreseeable injustices built in" and consequently privileges populations in the minority world (Moran-Thomas 2017). The glucometer points to larger inequalities within the global health arena, whereby medical resources may be found in abundance in some parts of the world, while they remain scarce in others. I used the glucometer as illustrative for the struggle to provide and maintain the most basic diagnostic access for diabetes. It raises the moral question of why some diseases are prioritized over others. Why is it justified to use the glucometer for diagnostic purposes in Uganda and elsewhere, while it would never be used for the diagnosis of diabetes in parts of the majority world? The glucometer hereby is not a technological device, which could not be changed or adjusted to also meet the needs for other settings (ibid., see also Akrich 1992) and there is movement going on. Pioneering projects intend to modify the glucometer so that it is suitable for diagnostic purposes and applicable also in settings with curtailed health infrastructures (see for instance Apkan 2015; Saha et al. 2014). But it is happening at a speed that does not match the scope of the problem.

Perhaps diabetes does not promise to become a success story that can be tackled with a "solution in a box" (Redfield 2012a). There will be no global answer to diabetes or other chronic conditions, but, as my research has shown, we need to develop global approaches, enabling local answers and solutions. Solutions that are adjusted to the given circumstances, resources and infrastructures available locally. If not, then the diagnosis of diabetes will continue to follow a logic of chance, and not be granted the human right like the access to basic health care ought to be. This is, without a doubt, a normative discussion, but it has an inevitable existential dimension, on which well-being and life depend. In this sense, I sympathize with Men et al. (2012) and their demand that the rising double burden of diseases calls for action among scholars, governments, international organizations, and national institutions to "move on from an understandable preoccupation with HIV/AIDS to address a range of chronic diseases [,] which are becoming the major cause of morbidity and mortality in many developing countries" (ibid.: 36). If the global health agenda does not start to appreciate the needs of chronic diseases such as diabetes, diabetes and other chronic diseases will continue to struggle for visibility.

References

Abramowitz, S.A. & Panter-Brick, C., 2015. *Medical humanitarianism: ethnographies of practice*, Philadelphia: University of Pennsylvania Press.

Adams, V., 2016. Metrics of the Global Sovereign: Numbers and Stories in Global Health. In V. Adams, ed. *Metrics. What Counts in Global Health*. Durham: Duke University Press, pp. 19–54.

Adams, V., 2013. Evidence-Based Global Public Health. In J. G. Biehl & A. Petryna, eds. *When People Come First*. Princeton, New Jersey: Princeton University Press, pp. 54–90.

Adams, V. & Biehl, J., 2016. The work of evidence in critical global health. *Medicine Anthropology Theory*, 3(2), pp. 123–126. Available at: https://pdfs.semanticscholar.org/4443/42730a01cfaa23e1916750bb074025fc0f9a.pdf [Accessed September 28, 2019].

Agarwal, R., Kalita, J.D. & Misra, U.D., 2008. Barriers to evidence based medicine practice in South Asia and possible solutions. *Neurology Asia*, 13, pp. 87–94. Available at: http://www.neurology-asia.org/articles/20082_087.pdf [Accessed September 28, 2019].

Akrich, M., 1993. Essay of Technosociology: A Gasogene in Costa Rica. In P. Lemonier, ed. *Technological choices. Transformation in material cultures since the Neolithic*. London: Routledge, pp. 289–337. Available at: https://halshs.archives-ouvertes.fr/halshs-00081732/document [Accessed September 28, 2019].

Akrich, M., 1992. The De-Scription of Technical Objects. In W. E. Bijker & J. Law, eds. *Shaping Technology/Building Society*. Cambridge, Massachusetts/ London: MIT Press, pp. 205–224.

Alberti, K.G.M.M. & Zimmet, P.Z., 1998. Definition, diagnosis and classification of diabetes mellitus and its complications. Part 1: diagnosis and classification of diabetes mellitus. Provisional report of a WHO Consultation. *Diabetic Medicine*, 15(7), pp.539–553. Available at: https://onlinelibrary.wiley.com/doi/abs/10.1002/%28SICI%291096-9136%28199807%2915%3A7%3C539%3A%3AAID-DIA668%3E3.0.CO%3B2-S. [Accessed September 28, 2019].

Al-Gelban, K.S. et al., 2009. Barriers against application of evidence-based medicine in general hospitals in Aseer region, kingdom of Saudi Arabia. *Journal of family & community medicine*, 16(1), pp. 1–5. Available at: http://www.ncbi.nlm. nih.gov/pubmed/23012182 [Accessed September 28, 2019].

Al-Lawati, J.A., 2017. Diabetes Mellitus: A Local and Global Public Health Emergency! *Oman medical journal*, 32(3), pp. 177–179. Available at: http://www.ncbi. nlm.nih.gov/pubmed/28584596 [Accessed September 28, 2019].

Allen, L.N. et al., 2017. What's in a name? A call to reframe non-communicable diseases. *The Lancet. Global health*, 5(2), pp. e129–e130. Available at: http://www. ncbi.nlm.nih.gov/pubmed/28104173 [Accessed September 12, 2019].

Allen, L.N. & Feigl, A.B., 2017. Reframing non-communicable diseases as socially transmitted conditions, pp. e644–e646. Available at: http://www.thelancet. com/pdfs/journals/langlo/PIIS2214-109X(17)30200-0.pdf [Accessed September 11, 2019].

American Diabetes Association (ADA), 2016. Classification and Diagnosis of Diabetes. *Diabetes Care*, 39(1), pp. 13–22. Available at: http://care.diabetesjournals. org/cgi/doi/10.2337/dc15-S005 [Accessed September 11, 2019].

American Diabetes Association (ADA), 2015. 2. Classification and Diagnosis of Diabetes. *Diabetes Care*, 38(1), pp. S8–S16. Available at: http://care.diabetesjournals. org/content/39/Supplement_1/S13 [Accessed September 11, 2019].

American Diabetes Association, 2011. Diagnosis and classification of diabetes mellitus. *Diabetes care*, 34 Suppl. 1, pp. S62-9. Available at: https://www.ncbi.nlm. nih.gov/pmc/articles/PMC3006051/ [Accessed September 11, 2019].

American Diabetes Association (ADA), 2004. Follow-up Report on the Diagnosis of Diabetes Mellitus. *Clinical Diabetes*, 22(2). Available at: http://clinical. diabetesjournals.org/content/22/2/71.short?patientinform-links=yes&legid= diaclin;22/2/71 [Accessed September 11, 2019].

Anderson, W., 2002. Introduction: Postcolonial Technoscience. *Social Studies of Science*, 32(5/6), pp. 643–658.

Andrews, N., Ernest Khalema, N. & Assié-Lumumba, N.T., 2015. *Millennium Development Goals (MDGs) in Retrospect. Africa's Development Beyond 2015*, Berlin, Heidelberg: Springer Verlag.

Armstrong, D., 1995. The rise of surveillance medicine. *Sociology of Health and Illness*, 17(3), pp. 393–404. Available at: http://doi.wiley.com/10.1111/1467-9566. ep10933329 [Accessed September 27, 2019].

Assah, F.K. & Mbanya, J.-C., 2009. Diabetes in Sub-Saharan Africa – Overview of a Looming Health Challenge. *European Endocrinology*, 5(0), p. 13. Available at: http://www.touchendocrinology.com/articles/diabetes-sub-saharan-africa-overview-looming-health-challenge-0 [Accessed September 27, 2019].

Bahendeka, S. et al., 2016. Prevalence and correlates of diabetes mellitus in Uganda: a population-based national survey. *Tropical Medicine & International Health*, 21(3), pp. 405–416. Available at: http://www.ncbi.nlm.nih.gov/pubmed/ 26729021 [Accessed September 22, 2019].

Balint, M., 2002. *The Doctor, His Patient and the Illness*, Madison, Connecticut: International Universities Press.

Barr, B., Bambra, C. & Smith, K.E., 2016. For the good of the cause: Generating evidence to inform social policies that reduce health inequalities. In K. E. Smith, S. Hill, & C. Bambra, eds. *Health Inequalities. Critical perspectives*. Oxford: Oxford University Press, pp. 252–264.

Baumstark, A. et al., 2017. Evaluation of Accuracy of Six Blood Glucose Monitoring Systems and Modeling of Possibly Related Insulin Dosing Errors. *Diabetes Technology & Therapeutics*, p.dia.2016.0408. Available at: http://online.liebertpub.com/doi/10.1089/dia.2016.0408 [Accessed September 22, 2019].

Beck, K., Klaeger, G. & Stasik, M., 2017. *The Making of the African Road*, Leiden: Brill My Book.

Beck, K., 2001. Die Aneignung der Maschine. In K.-H. Kohl & N. Schafhausen, eds. *New Heimat*. New York: Lukas & Sternberg, pp. 66–77.

Beisel, U., 2014. On gloves, rubber and the spatio-temporal logics of global health. *Somatosphere*, pp.1–5. Available at: http://somatosphere.net/2014/10/rubber-gloves-global-health.html [Accessed September 22, 2019].

Beisel, U. & Schneider, T., 2012. From 7/83-2 to Dr. JESUS: The transformation of a German ambulance car to a Ghanaian bus. *Environment and Planning D: Society and Space*, 30(4), pp. 639–654.

Benatar, S.R., Lister, G. & Thacker, S.C., 2010. Values in global health governance. *Global Public Health*, 5(2), pp. 143–153.

Berger, T. & Esguerra, A., 2017. *World Politics in Translation* T. Berger & A. Esguerra, eds., Abingdon: Taylor and Francis.

Bernard, H.R., 2011. *Research methods in anthropology: qualitative and quantitative approaches*, New York: AltaMira Press.

Biehl, J., 2012. Care and Disregard. In D. Fassin, ed. *A Companion to Moral Anthropology*. Malden, Oxford, Victoria: Wiley-Blackwell, pp. 242–263.

Biehl, J. & Petryna, A., 2014. Peopling global health. *Saude e Sociedade*, 23(2), pp. 376–389. Available at: www.scielo.br/pdf/sausoc/v23n2/0104-1290-sausoc-23-2-0376.pdf [Accessed September 22, 2019].

Biehl, J.G. & Petryna, A., 2013. *When people come first: critical studies in global health* J. G. Biehl & A. Petryna, eds., Princeton, New Jersey: Princeton University Press.

Black, W.C., 2000. Overdiagnosis: An underrecognized cause of confusion and harm in cancer screening. *Journal of the National Cancer Institute*, 92(16), pp. 1280–1282. Available at: https://www.ncbi.nlm.nih.gov/pubmed/10944539 [Accessed September 22, 2019].

Bliss, M., 2007. *The discovery of Insulin*, Chicago: University of Chicago Press.

Boruch, R. et al., 2017. Randomized controlled trials. In B. Greve, ed. *Handbook of Social Policy Evaluation*. Cheltenham: Edward Elgar Publishing Limited, pp. 15–37.

Boutayeb, A., 2006. The double burden of communicable and non-communicable diseases in developing countries. *Transactions of the Royal Society of Tropical Medicine and Hygiene*, 100(3), pp. 191–199.

Bowker, G.C. & Star, S.L., 1999. *Sorting things out: classification and its consequences*, Cambridge, Massachusetts/ London: MIT Press.

Bowker, G.C., 1995. Second Nature Once Removed. *Time & Society*, 4(1), pp. 47–66.

Bowker, G.C. et al., 2015. *Boundary objects and beyond: working with Leigh Star* G. C. Bowker et al., eds., Cambridge, Massachusetts/ London: MIT Press.

Brolan, C.E. et al., 2015. "Everywhere but not specifically somewhere": a qualitative study on why the right to health is not explicit in the post-2015 negotiations. *BMC international health and human rights*, 15, p. 22. Available at: http://www.ncbi.nlm.nih.gov/pubmed/26293324 [Accessed September 28, 2019].

Brown, H. & Prince, R.J., 2015. ASR Focus on Volunteer Labor in East Africa Introduction: Volunteer Labor—Pasts and Futures of Work, Development, and Citizenship in East Africa. *African Studies Association*, 58(2), pp. 29–42. Available at: https://www.cambridge.org/core/services/aop-cambridge-core/content/view/CC11E036B99D047DC2C5464F03A7A5DD/S0002020615000360a.pdf/introduction_volunteer_laborpasts_and_futures_of_work_development_and_citizenship_in_east_africa.pdf [Accessed September 26, 2019].

Brown, T.M., Cueto, M. & Fee, E., 2006. The World Health Organization and the transition from "International" to "Global" Public Health. *American journal of public health*, 96(1), pp. 62–72. Available at: http://www.ncbi.nlm.nih.gov/pubmed/16322464 [Accessed September 19, 2019].

Brownson, R.C. et al., 2017. *Evidence-Based Decision Making in Public Health* Third Edit., Oxford: Oxford University Press.

Bruni, A. & Rizzi, C., 2013. Looking for data in diabetes healthcare: Patient 2.0 and the re-engineering of clinical encounters. *Science and Technology Studies*, 26(2), pp. 29–43.

Bury, M., 1982. Chronic illness as biographical disruption. *Sociology of Health and Illness*, 4(2), pp. 167–182. Available at: http://doi.wiley.com/10.1111/1467-9566.ep11339939 [Accessed September 28, 2019].

Buse, K. & Hawkes, S., 2015. Health in the sustainable development goals: ready for a paradigm shift? *Globalization and Health*, 11(1), p. 13. Available at: http://www.globalizationandhealth.com/content/11/1/13 [Accessed September 11, 2019].

Bygbjerg, I.C., 2012. Double Burden of Noncommunicable and Infectious Diseases in Developing Countries. *Science*, 337(6101), pp. 1499–1501. Available at: http://www.sciencemag.org/cgi/doi/10.1126/science.1223466 [Accessed September 28, 2019].

Calkins, S. & Rottenburg, R., 2017. Evidence, infrastructure and worth. In *Infrastructures and social complexity: a companion* P. Harvey, C. B. Jensen, & A. Morita, eds., Abingdon: Routledge, Taylor & Francis Group.

Callon, M., 1986. Power, action and belief: a new sociology of knowledge? In J. Law, ed. *Some elements of a sociology of translation: domestication of the scallops and the fishermen of St Brieux Bay*. London: Routledge, pp. 196–223.

Campo, R., 2006. "Anecdotal evidence": Why narratives matter to medical practice. *PLoS Medicine*, 3(10), pp. 1677–1678.

Camus, A., 1955/ 1991. *The Myth Of Sisyphus And Other Essays*. New York: Vintage International.

Cartwright, E., Hardon, A. & Manderson, L., 2016. Ways of Caring. In E. Cartwright, A. Hardon, & L. Manderson, eds. *The Routledge Handbook of Medical Anthropology*. New York/ London: Routledge, pp. 164–182.

Casper, M.J. & Koenig, B.A., 1996. Reconfiguring Nature and Culture: Intersections of Medical Anthropology and Technoscience Studies. *Medical Anthropology Quarterly*, 10(4), pp. 523–536. Available at: http://www.jstor.org/stable/648660 [Accessed September 28, 2019].

Cassell, E.J., 1976. *The Healers Art: A new Approach to the Doctor-Patient relationship*, Harmondsworth: Penguin Books.

Chakrabarty, D., 2000. *Provincializing Europe*, Princeton: Princeton University Press.

Chambers, D.W. & Gillespie, R., 2000. Locality in the History of Science: Colonial Science, Technoscience, and Indigenous Knowledge. *Osiris*, 15, pp. 221–240. Available at: http://www.jstor.org/stable/301950 [Accessed September 28, 2019].

Chatterjee, S., Khunti, K. & Davies, M.J., 2017. Type 2 diabetes. *Lancet (London, England)*, 389(10085), pp.2239–2251. Available at: http://www.ncbi.nlm.nih.gov/pubmed/28190580 [Accessed September 28, 2019].

Chinnock, P., Siegfried, N. & Clarke, M., 2005. Is Evidence-Based Medicine Relevant to the Developing World? *PLoS Medicine*, 2(5), pp. 0367–0369. Available at: http://dx.plos.org/10.1371/journal.pmed.0020107 [Accessed September 28, 2019].

Clark, J., 2014. Medicalization of global health 1: has the global health agenda become too medicalized? *Global health action*, 7, p. 23998. Available at: http://www.ncbi.nlm.nih.gov/pubmed/24848659 [Accessed September 23, 2019].

Clarke, S.F. & Foster, J.R., 2012. A history of blood glucose meters and their role in self-monitoring of diabetes mellitus. *British Journal of Biomedical Science*, 69(2), pp. 83–93.

Clemens, M.A., Kenny, C.J. & Moss, T.J., 2007. The Trouble with the MDGs: Confronting Expectations of Aid and Development Success. Available at: http://faculty.ucr.edu/ jorgea/econ181/clemens_etal_wd07.pdf [Accessed September 28, 2019].

Cohen, J., 2006. The New World of Global Health. *Science*, 311(5758), pp. 162–167. Available at: http://www.ncbi.nlm.nih.gov/pubmed/16410496 [Accessed September 28, 2019].

Conalogue, D.M. et al., 2017. International consultation on long-term global health research priorities, research capacity and research uptake in developing countries. *Health Research Policy and Systems*, 15(24), pp. 1–6. Available at: http://health-policy-systems.biomedcentral.com/articles/10.1186/s12961-017-0181-0 [Accessed September 28, 2019].

Crane, J.T., 2013. *Scrambling for Africa: AIDS, Expertise, and the Rise of American Global Health Science*, Ithaca and London: Cornell University Press.

Crawford, J., 2017. *Spiritually-Engaged Knowledge: The Attentive Heart*, Abingdon: Routledge.

Crump, J.A. & Sugarman, J., 2008. Ethical considerations for short-term experiences by trainees in global health. *JAMA*, 300(12), pp. 1456–8. Available at: http://www.ncbi.nlm.nih.gov/pubmed/18812538 [Accessed September 28, 2019].

Czarniawska, B. & Sevón, G., 2005. *Global Ideas. How Ideas, Objects and Practices Travel in the Global Economy*, Copenhagen: Copenhagen Business School.

Czupryniak, L. et al., 2014. Self-monitoring of blood glucose in diabetes: from evidence to clinical reality in Central and Eastern Europe—recommendations from the international Central-Eastern European expert group. *Diabetes technology & therapeutics*, 16(7), pp. 460–75. Available at: http://www.ncbi.nlm.nih.gov/pubmed/24716890 [Accessed September 28, 2019].

Dave, M., 2016. Health for All. In N. Shawki, ed. *International Norms, Normative Change, and the UN Sustainable Development Goals*. Lanham: Lexington Books, p. 85-98.

Davidoff, F. et al., 1995. Evidence based medicine. *BMJ: British Medical Journal*, 310(6987), p. 1085.

Dehue, T., 2010. Comparing Artificial Groups: On the History and Assumptions of the Randomised Controlled Trial. In C. Will & T. Moreira, eds. *Medical Proofs, Social Experiments: Clinical Trials in Shifting Contexts*. Farnham and Burlington: Ashgate Publishing, pp. 103–119.

de Laet, M. & Mol, A., 2000. The Zimbabwe Bush Pump: Mechanics of a Fluid Technology. *Social Studies of Science*, 30, pp. 225–263.

de Laet, M., 2002. *Research in Science and Technology Studies: Knowledge and Technology Transfer* M. de Laet, ed., Amsterdam, Boston, London, New York, Oxford, Paris, San Diego, San Francisco, Singapore, Sydney, Tokyo: JAI, an imprint of Elsevier Science.

DelVecchio Good, M.-J., Good, B.J. & Grayman, J., 2010. Complex Engagements: Responding to Violence in Postconflict Aceh. In D. Fassin & M. Pandolfi, eds. *Contemporary States of Emergency: The Politics of Military and Humanitarian Interventions*. New York: Zone Books, pp. 241–268.

Diaz-Bone, R. & Didier, E., 2016. The sociology of quantification -perspectives on an emerging field in the social sciences. *Historical Social Research*, 41(2), pp. 7–26. Available at: http://www.ssoar.info/ssoar/bitstream/handle/document/

46872/ssoar-hsr-2016-2-diaz-bone_et_al-The_sociology_of_quantification_-.pdf?sequence=1 [Accessed September 29, 2019].

Dieleman, J., Murray, C.J.L. & Haakenstad, A., 2013. *Financing Global Health 2013: Transition in an Age of Austerity*, Seattle. Available at: http://www.healthdata.org/sites/default/files/files/policy_report/2014/FGH2013/IHME_FGH2013_Full_Report.pdf [Accessed September 29, 2019].

Dods, R.F., 2013. *Understanding diabetes: a biochemical perspective*, Hoboken, New Jersey: John Wiley & Sons, Ltd.

Easterly, W., 2009. How the Millennium Development Goals are Unfair to Africa. *World Development*, 37(1), pp. 26–35.

Ecks, S., 2009. Three propositions for an evidence-based anthropology. In M. Engelke, ed. *The objects of evidence: anthropological approaches to the production of knowledge*. Malden, Oxford, Victoria: Wiley-Blackwell, p. 74-88.

Eliasoph, N., 2011. *Making volunteers: civic life after welfare's end*, Princeton, New Jersey: Princeton University Press.

Engelhardt, D., 1989. *Diabetes. Its Medical and Cultural History*, Berlin Heidelberg: Springer Verlag.

Erikson, S.L., 2012. Global health business: the production and performativity of statistics in Sierra Leone and Germany. *Medical anthropology*, 31(4), pp.367–84. Available at: http://www.ncbi.nlm.nih.gov/pubmed/22746684 [Accessed September 29, 2019].

Espeland, W.N. & Stevens, M.L., 2008. A Sociology of Quantification. *European Journal of Sociology*, 49(3), p. 401.

Evans, M.L. & Amiel, S.A., 2002. Hypoglycemia. In J. A. H. Wass et al., eds. *Oxford Textbook of Endocrinology and Diabetes*. Oxford: Oxford University Press, pp. 1717–1725.

Falzon, M.-A., 2009. *Multi-sited Ethnography: Theory, Praxis and Locality in Contemporary Research*, Farnham and Burlington: Ashgate Publishing Limited.

Farmer, A. et al., 2009. Blood glucose self-monitoring in type 2 diabetes: a randomised controlled trial. *Health Technology Assessment*, 13(15), p. iii–iv, ix–xi, 1-50. Available at: http://www.ncbi.nlm.nih.gov/pubmed/19254484 [Accessed September 28, 2019].

Farmer, P., 2014. Diary. *London Review of Books*, 36(20), pp. 38–39. Available at: https://www.lrb.co.uk/v36/n20/paul-farmer/diary [Accessed September 28, 2019].

Fassin, D., 2012a. *A companion to moral anthropology*, Oxford: Wiley-Blackwell.

Fassin, D., 2012b. That Obscure Object of Global Health. In M. C. Inhorn & E. A. Wentzell, eds. *Medical Anthropology at the Intersections*. Durham: Duke University Press, pp. 95–115.

Feierman, S., 2017/ 2011. When Physicians Meet: Local Medical Knowledge. In W. Geissler & C. Molyneux, eds. *Evidence, Ethos and Experiment: The Anthropology and History of Medical Research in Africa*. New York: Berghahn Books, pp. 171–197.

Felt, U. et al., 2017. *The Handbook of Science and Technology Studies* 4th ed. U. Felt et al., eds., Cambridge, Massachusetts/ London: MIT Press.

Feudtner, J.C., 2003. *Bittersweet: diabetes, insulin, and the transformation of illness* A. M. Brandt & L. R. Churchill, eds., Chapel Hill & London: The University of North Carolina Press.

Fishman, J.R., Mamo, L. & Grzanka, P.R., 2017. Sex, Gender, and Sexuality in Biomedicine. In U. Felt et al., eds. *The Handbook of Science and Technology Studies*. Cambridge, Massachusetts, London: MIT Press, pp. 379–406.

Foucault, M., 1998. *Ethics: Subjectivity and Truth* P. Rabinow, ed., New York: The New Press.

Foucault, M., 1988. Technologies of the Self. In L. Martin, H. Gutman, & P. Hutton, eds. *Technologies of the Self: A Seminar with Michel Foucault*. London: Tavistock, pp. 16–49.

Foucault, M., 1986. *The care of the Self: The History of Sexuality: An Introduction*, vol.3. New York: Pantheon.

Foucault, M., 1979. *The History of Sexuality: An Introduction*. London: Penguin.

Freeman, R., 2009. What is "translation"? *Evidence & Policy*, 5(4), pp. 429–447.

Gill, G. V. et al., 2009. A sub-Saharan African perspective of diabetes. *Diabetologia*, 52(1), pp. 8–16.

Goldenberg, M.J., 2006. On evidence and evidence-based medicine: Lessons from the philosophy of science. *Social Science & Medicine*, 62, pp. 2621–2632. Available at: https://philpapers.org/archive/GOLOEA-2.pdf [Accessed September 28, 2019].

Jutel, A. & Dew, K., 2014. *Social Issues in Diagnosis. An Introduction for Students and Clinicians*, Baltimore, Maryland: Johns Hopkins University Press.

Gordon, D.R., 1988. Clinical Science and Clinical Expertise: Changing Boundaries between Art and Science in Medicine. In M. Lock & D. Gordon, eds. *Biomedicine Examined*. Dordrecht: Springer Netherlands, pp. 257–295.

Granado, S. et al., 2011. Appropriating "Malaria": Local Responses to Malaria Treatment and Prevention in Abidjan, Côte d'Ivoire. *Medical Anthropology*, 30(1), pp. 102–121.

Guell, C., 2012. Self-Care at the Margins: Meals and Meters in Migrants' Diabetes Tactics. *Medical Anthropology Quarterly*, 26(4), pp. 518–533.

Guell, C., 2009. *Tactics of Diabetes Control*. PhD-Thesis, The University of Edinburgh. Available at: https://www.era.lib.ed.ac.uk/bitstream/handle/1842/4293/Guell2009.pdf?sequence=2&isAllowed=y [Accessed September 28, 2019].

Hacking, I., 2002. *Historical Ontology*, Cambridge, Massachusetts: Harvard University Press.

Hadolt, B., Hörbst, V. & Müller-Rockstroh, B., 2012. Biomedical Techniques in Context: On the Appropriation of Biomedical Procedures and Artifacts. *Medical Anthropology*, 31(3), pp. 179–195.

Hahn, H.P., 2008. *Consumption in Africa: anthropological approaches*, Münster: LIT Verlag.

Han, P.K., 1997. Historical changes in the objectives of the periodic health examination. *Annals of internal medicine*, 127(10), pp. 910–917. Available at: http://www.ncbi.nlm.nih.gov/pubmed/9382370 [Accessed September 28, 2019].

Hannerz, U., 2003. Being there... and there... and there! *Ethnography*, 4(2), pp. 201–216.

Harding, S., 2009. Postcolonial and feminist philosophies of science and technology: convergences and dissonances. *Postcolonial Studies*, 12(4), pp. 401–421. Available at: http://www.tandfonline.com/doi/full/10.1080/13688790903350658 [Accessed September 28, 2019].

Hardon, A. 2016. Testing Pregnant Women for HIV. Contestations in the Global Effort to Reduce the Spread of AIDS. In *Diagnostic Controversy. Cultural Perspectives on Competing Knowledge in Healthcare*. Abingdon: Routledge, Taylor & Francis Group, pp. 27-46.

Hardon, A. & Moyer, E., 2014. Medical technologies: flows, frictions and new socialities. *Anthropology & Medicine*, 21(2), pp. 107–112.

Harvey, P., Jensen, C.B. & Morita, A., 2017. *Infrastructures and social complexity: a companion* P. Harvey, C. B. Jensen, & A. Morita, eds., Abingdon: Routledge, Taylor & Francis Group.

Hawkes, C. & Popkin, B.M., 2015. Can the sustainable development goals reduce the burden of nutrition-related non-communicable diseases without truly addressing major food system reforms? *BMC medicine*, 13(1), p. 143. Available at: http://www.biomedcentral.com/1741-7015/13/143 [Accessed September 28, 2019].

Hawkins, R.C., 2005. The Evidence Based Medicine approach to diagnostic testing: practicalities and limitations. *The Clinical biochemist. Reviews*, 26(2), pp. 7–18. Available at: http://www.ncbi.nlm.nih.gov/pubmed/16278748 [Accessed September 28, 2019].

Hayford, JT, Weydert, J. & Thompson, R., 1983. Validity of Urine Glucose Measurements for Estimating Plasma Glucose Concentration. *Diabetes care*, 4(1), pp. 40–44.

Herman, W.H. & Zimmet, P., 2012. Type 2 Diabetes: An Epidemic Requiring Global Attention and Urgent Action. *Diabetes Care*, 35(5), pp. 943–944. Available at: http://care.diabetesjournals.org/content/35/5/943 [Accessed September 23, 2019].

Heurtin-Roberts, S. & Becker, G., 1993. Anthropological perspectives on chronic illness. Introduction. *Social science & medicine (1982)*, 37(3), pp. 281–283. Available at: http://www.ncbi.nlm.nih.gov/pubmed/8356477 [Accessed September 25, 2019].

Hilton, M. & McKay, J., 2011. *The ages of voluntarism: how we got to the Big Society*, Oxford: Oxford University Press.

Hjelm, K. & Atwine, F., 2011. Health-care seeking behaviour among persons with diabetes in Uganda: an interview study. *BMC International Health and Human Rights*, 11(1), p.11. Available at: http://www.biomedcentral.com/1472-698X/11/11 [Accessed September 25, 2019].

Hsu, E. & Potter, C., 2015. *Medical anthropology in Europe: shaping the Field*, Abingdon: Routledge.

International Diabetes Federation (IDF), 2015. *IDF Diabetes Atlas* 7th edn., Brussels: International Diabetes Federation. Available at: http://www.diabetesatlas.org [Accessed September 28, 2019].

International Diabetes Federation (IDF), 2009. *Guideline Self-Monitoring of Blood Glucose in Non-Insulin Treated Type 2 Diabetes*, Brussels. Available at: www.idf.org and at www.smbg-iwg.com [Accessed September 28, 2019].

International Diabetes Federation (IDF), 2008. *International Diabetes Federation (IDF), Africa Regional Meeting Implementation of the United Nations Resolution on Diabetes (61/225) in Africa, 19 December 2008, Nairobi, Kenya.*

Janssens, B. et al., 2007. Offering integrated care for HIV/AIDS, diabetes and hypertension within chronic disease clinics in Cambodia. *Bulletin of the World Health Organization*, 85(11), pp. 880–885. Available at: http://www.ncbi.nlm.nih.gov/pubmed/18038079 [Accessed September 19, 2019].

Johnson, J.L. et al., 2017. Barriers to Patient Use of Control Solution for Glucose Meters: Surveys of Patients, Pharmacists, and Providers in a Metropolitan Area. *Journal of Diabetes Science and Technology*, 11(3), pp. 553–557. Available at: http://journals.sagepub.com/doi/10.1177/1932296816678427 [Accessed September 28, 2019].

Jutel, A., 2011. *Putting a name to it. Diagnosis in contemporary society*, Baltimore, Maryland: Johns Hopkins University Press.

Jutel, A., 2009. Sociology of diagnosis: a preliminary review. *Sociology of Health & Illness*, 31(2), pp. 278–299. Available at: http://doi.wiley.com/10.1111/j.1467-9566.2008.01152.x [Accessed September 28, 2019].

Kelly, A., 2010. Pragmatic Fact-making: Contracts and Contexts in the UK and the Gambia. In C. Will & T. Moreira, eds. *Medical Proofs, Social Experiments: Clinical Trials in Shifting Contexts*. Farnham and Burlington: Ashgate Publishing, pp. 121–136.

Kerner, W., 2001. Definition, Klassifikation und Diagnostik des Diabetes Mellitus. In W. A. Scherbaum, K. W. Lauterbach, & H. G. Josst, eds. *Evidenzbasierte Diabetes. Leitlinien DDG*. Deutsche Diabetes Gesellschaft.

King, H. et al., 1991. Update / Le point Diabetes in adults is now a Third World problem. *Europe*, pp. 643–648.

Kirk, J.K. & Stegner, J., 2010. Self-monitoring of blood glucose: practical aspects. *Journal of diabetes science and technology*, 4(2), pp. 435–439. Available at: http://www.ncbi.nlm.nih.gov/pubmed/20307405 [Accessed September 28, 2019].

Klonoff, D.C. & Prahalad, P., 2015. Performance of Cleared Blood Glucose Monitors. *Journal of Diabetes Science and Technology*, 9(4), pp. 895–910. Available at: http://www.ncbi.nlm.nih.gov/pubmed/25990294 [Accessed September 28, 2019].

Klonoff, D.C., 2008. New evidence demonstrates that self-monitoring of blood glucose does not improve outcomes in type 2 diabetes-when this practice is not applied properly. *Journal of diabetes science and technology*, 2(3), pp. 342–348. Available at: http://www.ncbi.nlm.nih.gov/pubmed/19885197 [Accessed September 28, 2019].

Knaapen, L., 2014. Evidence-Based Medicine or Cookbook Medicine? Addressing Concerns over the Standardization of Care. *Sociology Compass*, 8(6), pp. 823–836. Available at: https://onlinelibrary.wiley.com/doi/abs/10.1111/soc4.12184 [Accessed September 28, 2019].

Koch, E., 2016. Resisting Tuberculosis or TB Resistance. Enacting Diagnosis in Georgian Labs and Prisons. In *Diagnostic Controversy. Cultural Perspectives on Competing Knowledge in Healthcare*. Abingdon: Routledge, Taylor & Francis Group, pp. 47–75.

Kohn, M.A., 2014. Understanding evidence-based diagnosis. *Diagnosis*, 1(1), pp. 39–42. Available at: https://www.degruyter.com/view/j/dx.2014.1.issue-1/dx-2013-0003/dx-2013-0003.xml [Accessed September 28, 2019].

Koplan, J.P. et al., 2009. Towards a common definition of global health. *Lancet (London, England)*, 373(9679), pp. 1993–1995. Available at: http://www.ncbi.nlm.nih.gov/pubmed/19493564 [Accessed September 28, 2019].

Kuhanen, J., 2008. The Historiography of HIV and AIDS in Uganda. *History in Africa*, 35, pp. 301–325.

Lakoff, A., 2010. Two Regimes of Global Health. *Humanity: An International Journal of Human Rights, Humanitarianism, and Development*, 1(1), pp. 59–79. Available at: http://muse.jhu.edu/content/crossref/journals/humanity/v001/1.1.lakoff.html [Accessed September 28, 2019].

Lakoff, A. & Collier, S.J., 2008. *Biosecurity Interventions: Global Health and Security in Question*, New York: Columbia University Press.

Lambert, H., 2009. Evidentiary truths? The evidence of anthropology through the anthropology of medical evidence. *Anthropology Today*, 25(1), pp. 16–20. Available at: http://onlinelibrary.wiley.com/doi/10.1111/j.1467-8322.2009.00642.x/abstract [Accessed September 28, 2019].

Lampland, M. & Star, S.L., 2009. *Standards and their stories: how quantifying, classifying, and formalizing practices shape everyday life*, New York and London: Cornell University Press.

Larkin, B., 2013. The Politics and Poetics of Infrastructure. *Annual Review of Anthropology*, 42(1), pp. 327–343. Available at: http://www.annualreviews.org/doi/10.1146/annurev-anthro-092412-155522 [Accessed September 28, 2019].

Latour, B., 2005. *Reassembling the Social. An Introduction to Actor-Network-Theory*, New York: Oxford University Press.

Latour, B., 1987. *Science in action: how to follow scientists and engineers through society*, Cambridge, Massachusetts: Harvard University Press.

Latour, B., 1986/z1999. The powers of association. In Law, John: Power, action, and belief: a new sociology of knowledge? *Sociological review monograph*; 32, p. 264–280.

Lhachimi, S.K., Bala, M.M. & Vanagas, G., 2016. Evidence-Based Public Health. *BioMed research international*, 2016, p. 1–2. Available at: http://www.ncbi.nlm.nih.gov/pubmed/26942196 [Accessed September 28, 2019].

Liebow, E. et al., 2013. On Evidence and the Public Interest. *American Anthropologist*, 115(4), pp. 642–655. Available at: http://doi.wiley.com/10.1111/aman.12053 [Accessed September 28, 2019].

Liggins, A.S. & Beisel, U., 2017. Translating the glucometer – from "Western" markets to Uganda: glucometer graveyards, missing testing strips and the difficulties of patient care. In *World Politics in Translation: Power, Relationality and Difference in Global Cooperation*. Abingdon: Taylor & Francis, pp. 59–75.

Lindelöw, M., Reinikka, R. & Svensson, J., 2003. *Health care on the frontlines: survey evidence on public and private providers in Uganda*, World Bank. Available at: http://agris.fao.org/agris-search/search.do?recordID=US2012407030 [Accessed September 28, 2019].

Lopez, A.D. et al., 2014. Remembering the forgotten non-communicable diseases. *BMC Medicine*, 12(1), p. 200. Available at: http://bmcmedicine.biomedcentral.com/articles/10.1186/s12916-014-0200-8 [Accessed September 28, 2019].

Lorenz, N., 2007. Effectiveness of global health partnerships: will the past repeat itself? *Bulletin of the World Health Organization*, 85(7), pp. 567–568. Available at: http://www.ncbi.nlm.nih.gov/pubmed/17768507 [Accessed September 28, 2019].

Lovrenčić, M.V. et al., 2013. Validation of Point-of-Care Glucose Testing for Diagnosis of Type 2 Diabetes. *International journal of endocrinology*, 2013. Available at: http://www.ncbi.nlm.nih.gov/pubmed/24382960 [Accessed September 28, 2019].

Lupton, D., 2016. *The Quantified Self*, Cambridge: Polity Press.

Lupton, D., 2001. The diagnostic test and the danger within. In M. Purdy & D. Banks, eds. *The Sociology and politics of health. A Reader*. London: Routledge, pp. 151–158.

Lupton, D., 1995. *The Imperative of Health. Public Health and the Regulated Body*, London: SAGE Publications Ltd.

Lynch, R. & Cohn, S., 2016. In the loop: Practices of self-monitoring from accounts by trial participants. *Health: An Interdisciplinary Journal for the Social Study of Health, Illness and Medicine*, 20(5), pp.523–538. Available at: http://journals.sagepub.com/doi/10.1177/1363459315611939 [Accessed September 28, 2019].

Macamo, E. & Neubert, D., 2008. The New and Its Temptations. Products of Modernity and Their Impact on Social Change in Africa. In A. Adogame, M. Echtler, & U. Vierke, eds. *Unpacking the New. Rethinking Cultural Syncretization in Africa and Beyond*. Münster: LIT Verlag, pp. 271–303.

Malinowski, B., 1984 [1922]. *Argonauts of the Western Pacific*, London: Routledge and Kegan Paul.

Manderson, L., Cartwright, E. & Hardon, A., 2016. *The Routledge Handbook of Medical Anthropology* L. Manderson, E. Cartwright, & A. Hardon, eds., New York/London: Routledge, Taylor & Francis Group.

Manderson, L. et al., 2010. *Chronic conditions, fluid states: chronicity and the anthropology of illness* L. Manderson & C. Smith-Morris, eds., New Brunswick, New Jersey: Rutgers University Press.

Marcus, G.E., 1995. Ethnography in/of the World System: The Emergence of Multi-Sited Ethnography. *Annual Review of Anthropology*, 24, pp. 95–117. Available at: http://www.dourish.com/classes/readings/Marcus-MultiSitedEthnography-ARA.pdf [Accessed September 28, 2019].

Marrero, S.L., Bloom, D.E. & Adashi, E.Y., 2012. Noncommunicable Diseases. *JAMA*, 307(19), pp. 876–878. Available at: http://jama.jamanetwork.com/article.aspx?doi=10.1001/jama.2012.3546 [Accessed September 28, 2019].

Marshall, S.J., 2004. Developing countries face double burden of disease. *Bulletin of the World Health Organization*, 82(7), p. 556. Available at: http://www.ncbi.nlm.nih.gov/pubmed/15500291 [Accessed September 28, 2019].

Mayega, R.W., 2014. *Prevalence, risk factors, perceptions and implications for the health system*. PhD-thesis, Makerere University and Stockholm University.

Maynard, R., 2010. Chronic conditions, fluid states: Chronicity and the anthropology of illness. In L. Manderson & C. M. Smith-Morris, eds. *Chronic Conditions, Fluid States: Chronicity and the Anthropology of Illness*. New Jersey: Rutgers University Press.

McEwan, C., 2001. Postcolonialism, feminism and development: intersections and dilemmas. *Progress in Development Studies*, 1(2), pp. 93–111. Available at: https://journals.sagepub.com/doi/10.1177/146499340100100201 [Accessed September 28, 2019].

Medjedovic, I. & Witzel, A., 2010. Wiederverwendung qualitativer Daten, Wiesbaden: VS Verlag.

Medvei, V.C., 1993. *The History of Clinical Endocrinology: A Comprehensive Account of Endocrinology from Earlies Times to the Present Day*, New York: Parthenon Publishing.

Meessen, B. et al., 2006. Poverty and user fees for public health care in low-income countries: lessons from Uganda and Cambodia. *The Lancet*, 368(9554), pp. 2253–2257.

Men, C. et al., 2012. "I Wish I Had AIDS": A qualitative study on access to health care services for HIV/AIDS and diabetic patients in Cambodia. *Health, Culture and Society*, 2(1), pp. 22–39. Available at: http://hcs.pitt.edu/ojs/index.php/hcs/article/view/67 [Accessed September 28, 2019].

Merriam-Webster, 2017. "Diagnosis." Available at: https://www.merriam-webster.com/dictionary/diagnosis [Accessed September 28, 2019].

Merry, S.E., 2016. *The Seductions of Quantification: Measuring Human Rights, Gender Violence, and Sex Trafficking*, Chicago and London: The University of Chicago Press.

Milligan, C. & Conradson, D., 2006. *Landscapes of voluntarism: new spaces of health, welfare and governance*, Bristol: Policy Press.

Mindry, D., 2001. Nongovernmental Organizations, "Grassroots" and the Politics of Virtue. *Signs*, 26(4), pp. 1187–1211.

Ministry of Health Uganda (MoH), 2016. *Non-Communicable Disease Risk Factor Baseline Survey Uganda 2014 Report*, Kampala. Available at: http://www.who.int/chp/steps/Uganda_2014_STEPS_Report.pdf [Accessed September 28, 2019].

Ministry of Health Uganda (MoH), 2015. *Health Sector Development Plan 2015/16-2019-20*, Kampala. Available at: https://www.google.de/url?sa=t&rct=j&q=&esrc=s&source=web&cd=1&cad=rja&uact=8&ved=0ahUKEwjDhrzsjqDWAhVIvRoKHS5jCboQFggmMAA&url=http%3A%2F%2Fhealth.go.ug%2Fdownload%2Ffile%2Ffid%2F834&usg=AFQjCNEg6ZHR2ugU5xwoXIAkLlw-P8wSjg [Accessed September 28, 2019].

Ministry of Health Uganda (MoH), 2014. *Uganda Hospital and Health Centre IV Census Survey*, Kampala. Available at: http://health.go.ug/sites/default/files/Hospital Census Report Jan 2016.pdf [Accessed September 28, 2019].

Mirowsky, J., Ross, C., 1989. Psychiatric diagnosis as reified measurement. *Journal of Health and Social Behavior*, 30 (1): pp. 11–40.

Mittermaier, A., 2014. Beyond compassion: Islamic voluntarism in Egypt. *American Ethnologist*, 41(3), pp. 518–531. Available at: http://doi.wiley.com/10.1111/amet.12092 [Accessed September 28, 2019].

Mol, A., Moser, I. & Pols, J., 2010. *Care in Practice: On Tinkering in Clinics, Homes and Farms*, Bielefeld: transcript Verlag.

Mol, A., 2008. *The logic of care*, New York/Abingdon, Oxon: Routledge.

Mol, A., 2002. *The Body Multiple: Ontology in Medical Practice*, Durham and London: Duke University Press.

Mol, A., 2000. What diagnostic devices do: The case of blood sugar measurement. *Theoretical Medicine and Bioethics*, 21(1), pp. 9–22.

Moore, A. & Stilgoe, J., 2009. Experts and Anecdotes: The Role of Anecdotal Evidence" in Public Scientific Controversies. *Science, Technology & Human Values*, 34(5), pp. 654–677. Available at: http://sth.sagepub.com/cgi/doi/10.1177/0162243908329382 [Accessed September 28, 2019].

Moran-Thomas, A., 2017. Glucometer foils. *Limn*. Available at: http://limn.it/glucometer-foils/.

Moretti, V., 2016. Dealing with numbers. Looking beyond the self-monitoring for a new technology of the self. *EASST Review*, 4(35). Available at: https://easst.net/article/dealing-with-numbers-looking-beyond-the-self-monitoring-for-a-new-technology-of-the-self/ [Accessed September 28, 2019].

Morrish, N.J. et al., 2001. Mortality and causes of death in the WHO Multinational Study of Vascular Disease in Diabetes. *Diabetologia*, 44 Suppl. 2(OCTOBER), pp. S14–S21. Available at: http://www.ncbi.nlm.nih.gov/pubmed/11587045 [Accessed September 28, 2019].

Muehlebach, A.K., 2012. *The moral neoliberal: welfare and citizenship in Italy*, Chicago: University of Chicago Press.

Müller-Rockstroh, B., 2007. *Ultrasound Travels The politics of a medical technology in Ghana and Tanzania*. PhD-thesis, Universitaire Pers Maastricht. Available at: https://cris.maastrichtuniversity.nl/portal/files/608185/guid-55791fcb-9886-4bd1-997f-4d98625f1c82-ASSET1.0 [Accessed September 28, 2019].

Murad, M.H. et al., 2016. New evidence pyramid. *Evidence Based Medicine*. Available at: http://ebm.bmj.com/content/early/2016/06/23/ebmed-2016-110401.abstract [Accessed September 28, 2019].

Nelkin, D. & Tancredi, L., 1994. *Dangerous Diagnostics: The Social Power of Biological Information* 2nd ed., Chicago: University of Chicago Press.

Neyland, D., 2013. An Ethnography of Numbers. In D. D. Caulkins & A. T. Jordan, eds. *A Companion to Organizational Anthropology*. Malden, Oxford, Victoria: Wiley-Blackwell, pp. 219–235.

Nielsen, A.J., 2010. *Traveling technologies and transformations in health care*, PhD series 36.2010, Copenhagen. Available at: http://openarchive.cbs.dk/bitstream/handle/10398/8212/Annegrete_Juul_Nielsen.pdf?sequence=1 [Accessed September 28, 2019].

Nielsen, M. & Grøn, L., 2013. Quantify Your Self! Numbers in Ambiguous Borderlands of Health. *Tidsskrift for Forskning i Sygdom og Samfund*, (19), pp. 55–74.

Nnko, S. et al., 2015. Chronic diseases in North-West Tanzania and Southern Uganda. Public perceptions of terminologies, aetiologies, symptoms and preferred management. *PLoS ONE*, 10(11).

O'Reilly, M. et al., 2010. "Dead in bed": A tragic complication of type 1 diabetes mellitus. *Irish Journal of Medical Science*, 179(4), pp. 585–587.

Omoleke, S.A., 2013. Chronic Non-Communicable Disease as a New Epidemic in Africa: Focus on The Gambia. *Pan African Medical Journal*, 14(1). Available at: http://www.panafrican-med-journal.com/content/article/14/87/full/ [Accessed September 28, 2019].

Oni-Orisan, A., 2016. The Obligation to Count: The Politics of Monitoring Maternal Mortality in Nigeria. In V. Adams, ed. *Metrics. What Counts in Global Health*. Durham: Duke University Press, pp. 82–101.

Onzivua, S., 2016. Wrong diagnosis lands doctor in jail. *Daily Monitor*. Available at: http://www.monitor.co.ug/artsculture/Reviews/Wrong-diagnosis-doctor-jail/691232-3480400-wtljvbz/index.html [Accessed September 28, 2019].

Papaspyros, N.S., 1964. *The History of Diabetes Mellitus*, Stuttgart: Georg Thieme Verlag.

Paxson, H., 2017. Participant-Observation and Interviewing Techniques. In J. Chrzan & J. Brett, eds. *Food Culture: Anthropology, Linguistics and Food Studies*. New York: Berghahn Books, pp. 92–100.

Pérez, R.L., 2017. Participant-Observation and Interviewing Techniques. In J. Chrzan & J. Brett, eds. *Food Culture: Anthropology, Linguistics and Food Studies*. New York: Berghahn Books, pp. 101–111.

Petrisor, B. & Bhandari, M., 2007. The hierarchy of evidence: Levels and grades of recommendation. *Indian journal of orthopaedics*, 41(1), pp. 11–15. Available at: http://www.ncbi.nlm.nih.gov/pubmed/21124676 [Accessed September 28, 2019].

Petryna, A., 2009. *When experiments travel: clinical trials and the global search for human subjects*, Princeton and Oxford: Princeton University Press.

Pinch, T., 2010. *On making infrastructure visible: Putting the non-humans to rights*. Cambridge Journal of Economy 34(1): pp. 77–89.

Powdermaker, H., 1966. *Stranger and friend: the way of an anthropologist*, New York: W.W. Norton.

Pollock, A. & Subramaniam, B., 2016. Resisting Power, Retooling Justice. *Science, Technology, & Human Values*, 41(6), pp. 951–966. Available at: http://journals.sagepub.com/doi/10.1177/0162243916657879 [Accessed September 28, 2019].

Poretsky, L. et al., 2010. *Principles of diabetes mellitus*, Berlin, Heidelberg: Springer Verlag.

Prince, R.J., 2014. Situating Health and the Public in Africa. In R. J. Prince & R. Marsland, eds. *Making and Unmaking Public Health in Africa*. Athens/ Ohio: Ohio University Press, pp. 1–51.

Puska, P., 2011. Non-communicable diseases – neglected diseases in global health work? *European journal of public health*, 21(3), p. 269.

Redfield, P., 2013. *Life in crisis: the ethical journey of Doctors without Borders*, Oakland: University of California Press.

Redfield, P., 2012a. Humanitarianism. In D. Fassin, ed. *A Companion to Moral Anthropology*. Hoboken, New Jersey: Wiley-Blackwell, pp. 451–467.

Redfield, P., 2012b. THE UNBEARABLE LIGHTNESS OF EX-PATS: Double Binds of Humanitarian Mobility. *Cultural Anthropology*, 27(2), pp. 358–382. Available at: http://doi.wiley.com/10.1111/j.1548-1360.2012.01147.x [Accessed September 28, 2019].

Redfield, P., 2008. Vital Mobility and the Humanitarian Kit. In S. J. Collier & A. Lakoff, eds. *Biosecurity Interventions. Global Health & Security in Question*. New York: Columbia University Press, pp. 147–171.

Redfield, P. & Bornstein, E., 2010. *Forces of compassion: humanitarianism between ethics and politics*, Santa Fe: School for Advanced Research Press.

Robben, A.C.G.M. & Sluka, J.A., 2007. *Ethnographic Fieldwork: An Anthropological Reader*, Malden, Oxford, Victoria: Wiley-Blackwell.

Rodriguez-Fernandez, R. et al., 2016. The double burden of disease among mining workers in Papua, Indonesia: at the crossroads between Old and New health paradigms. *BMC Public Health*, 16(951), pp. 1–7. Available at: http://bmcpublichealth.biomedcentral.com/articles/10.1186/s12889-016-3630-8 [Accessed September 28, 2019].

Roglic, G. et al., 2005. The burden of mortality attributable to diabetes: realistic estimates for the year 2000. *Diabetes care*, 28(9), pp. 2130–2135. Available at: http://www.ncbi.nlm.nih.gov/pubmed/16123478 [Accessed September 28, 2019].

Rosner, F., 1997. *The Medical Legacy of Moses Maimonides*, New Jersey: Ktav Pub Inc.

Rottenburg, R., 2015. *The world of indicators: the making of governmental knowledge through quantification*, Cambridge: Cambridge University Press.

Rottenburg, R., 2009. *Far-fetched facts: a parable of development aid*, Cambridge, Massachusetts/ London: MIT Press.

Sackett, D., 2000. Evidence-based medicine: how to practice and teach EBM. *Journal of Clinical Pathology*, 55(6), pp. 435–439. Available at: http://www.ncbi.nlm.nih.gov/pubmed/12037026 [Accessed September 28, 2019].

Sackett, D.L. et al., 1996. Evidence based medicine: what it is and what it isn't. *British medical journal*, 312(7023), pp. 71–72. Available at: http://www.ncbi.nlm.nih.gov/pmc/articles/PMC2349778/pdf/bmj00524-0009.pdf [Accessed September 28, 2019].

Sacks, D.B. et al., 2011. Guidelines and recommendations for laboratory analysis in the diagnosis and management of diabetes mellitus. *Diabetes care*, 34(6), pp. e61–e99. Available at: http://www.ncbi.nlm.nih.gov/pubmed/21617108 [Accessed September 28, 2019].

Saha, S., Sarker, N. & Hira, A., 2014. Design & implementation of a low cost blood glucose meter with high accuracy. In *2014 International Conference on Electrical En-*

gineering and Information & Communication Technology. IEEE, pp. 1–6. Available at: http://ieeexplore.ieee.org/lpdocs/epic03/wrapper.htm?arnumber=6919050 [Accessed September 28, 2019].

Saquib, N., Saquib, J. & Ioannidis, J.P., 2015. Does screening for disease save lives in asymptomatic adults? Systematic review of meta-analyses and randomized trials. *International Journal of Epidemiology*, 44(1), pp. 264–277. Available at: https://academic.oup.com/ije/article-lookup/doi/10.1093/ije/dyu140 [Accessed September 28, 2019].

Scandlyn, J., 2000. When AIDS became a chronic disease. *The Western journal of medicine*, 172(2), pp. 130–133. Available at: http://www.ncbi.nlm.nih.gov/pubmed/10693378 [Accessed September 28, 2019].

Seth, S., 2009. Putting knowledge in its place: science, colonialism, and the postcolonial. *Postcolonial Studies*, 12(4), pp. 373–388. Available at: http://www.tandfonline.com/doi/full/10.1080/13688790903350633 [Accessed September 28, 2019].

Shapin, S. & Schaffer, S., 2011/1986. *Leviathan and the air-pump: Hobbes, Boyle, and the experimental life: with a new introduction by the authors*, Princeton, New Jersey: Princeton University Press.

Sheridan, D.J., 2012. *Medical Science in the 21st Century: Sunset or New Dawn?*, London: Imperial College Press.

Simone, A., 2004. People as Infrastructure: Intersecting Fragments in Johannesburg. *Public Culture*, 16(3), pp. 407–429. Available at: http://publicculture.dukejournals.org/cgi/reprint/16/3/407 [Accessed September 28, 2019].

Smith-Morris, C.M., 2016. When Numbers and Stories Collide: Randomized Controlled Trials and the Search for Ethnographic Fidelity in the Veterans Administration. In V. Adams, ed. *Metrics. What Counts in Global Health*. Durham: Duke University Press, pp. 181–202.

Smith-Morris, C.M., 2015. *Diagnostic controversy: cultural perspectives on competing knowledge in healthcare*, London: Routledge.

Spittler, G., 2002. Globale Waren-lokale Aneignungen. In B. Hauser-Schäublin & U. Braukämper, eds. *Ethnologie der Globalisierung. Perspektiven kultureller Verflechtungen*. Berlin: Dietrich Reimer Verlag, pp. 15–30.

Srinivas, M., Sridher, N. & Umesh, J., 2016. Diabetic Ketoacidosis in Children: A Systematic Review. *Journal of Chalmeda Anand Rao Institute of Medical Sciences ISSN*, 11(1), pp. 30–41. Available at: http://caims.org/assets/journal/2016/CAIMS Journal__06.PDF [Accessed September 28, 2019].

Star, S. & Ruhleber, K., 1996. Steps Toward Design an Ecology and Access of Infrastructure: for Large Spaces Information. *Information Systems Research*, 7(1), pp. 111–134.

Star, S., 1999. The ethnography of infrastructure. American Behavioral Scientist 43(3): 377–391.

Street, A. et al., 2014. Diagnostics for Development. *Somatosphere*. Available at: http://somatosphere.net/2014/05/diagnostics-for-development.html [Accessed September 28, 2019].

Street, A., 2014a. Rethinking Infrastructures for Global Health. Lecture/ University of Edinburgh. Available at: https://www.youtube.com/watch?v=HehA7XmUzHM.

Street, A., 2014b. Rethinking Infrastructures for Global Health: A View from West Africa and Papua New Guinea. *Somatosphere*, pp. 1–5. Available at: http://somatosphere.net/?p=9591 [Accessed September 28, 2019].

Street, A., 2014c. *Biomedicine in an Unstable Place*, Durham: Duke University Press.

Subramaniam, B. et al., 2017. Feminism, Postcolonialism, Technoscience. In U. Felt et al., eds. *The Handbook of Science and Technology Studies*. Cambridge, Massachusetts/ London: MIT Press, pp. 407–433.

Tabish, S.A., 2007. Is Diabetes Becoming the Biggest Epidemic of the Twenty-first Century? *International journal of health sciences*, 1(2), pp. V–VIII. Available at: http://www.ncbi.nlm.nih.gov/pubmed/21475425 [Accessed September 28, 2019].

Tichenor, M., 2016. The Power of Data: Global Malaria Governance and the Senegalese Data Retention Strike. In V. Adams, ed. *Metrics. What Counts in Global Health*. Durham: Duke University Press, pp. 105–124.

Tilley, H., 2011. *Africa as a living laboratory: empire, development, and the problem of scientific knowledge, 1870-1950*, Chicago: University of Chicago Press.

Timmermans, S. & Berg, M., 2003. *The Gold Standard: The Challenge Of Evidence-Based Medicine*, Philadelphia: Temple University Press.

Timmermans, S. & Kolker, E.S., 2004. Evidence-Based Medicine and the Reconfiguration of Medical Knowledge. *Journal of Health and Social Behavior*, 45, pp. 177–193. Available at: https://www.jstor.org/stable/pdf/3653831.pdf?seq=1#page_scan_tab_contents [Accessed September 28, 2019].

Timmermans, S. & Mauck, A., 2005. The promises and pitfalls of evidence-based medicine. *Health affairs (Project Hope)*, 24(1), pp. 18–28. Available at: http://content.healthaffairs.org/content/24/1/18.abstract [Accessed September 28, 2019].

Tonyushkina, K. & Nichols, J.H., 2009. Glucose Meters: A Review of Technical Challenges to Obtaining Accurate Results. *Journal of Diabetes Science and Technology J Diabetes Sci Technol J Diabetes Sci Technol*, 33(4), pp. 971–980. Available at: https://www.ncbi.nlm.nih.gov/pmc/articles/PMC2769957/pdf/dst-03-0971.pdf [Accessed September 28, 2019].

Torgerson, D.J. & Torgerson, C.J., 2008. *Designing Randomised Trials in Health, Education and the Social Sciences: An Introduction*, New York: Palgrave Macmillan.

Turner, J.R., 2013. Hierarchy of Evidence. In M. D. Gellman & J. R. Turner, eds. *Encyclopedia of Behavioral Medicine*. New York, NY: Springer New York, pp. 963–964.

Uganda Bureau of Statistics (UBOS), 2017. *Uganda Demographic and Health Survey 2016. Key Indicators*, Kampala. Available at: http://health.go.ug/sites/default/files/Demographic and Health Survey.pdf [Accessed September 28, 2019].

Uganda Bureau of Statistics (UBOS), 2014. *National Population and Housing Census 2014*, Kampala. Available at: http://www.ubos.org/onlinefiles/uploads/ubos/NPHC/NPHC%202014%20PROVISIONAL%20RESULTS%20REPORT.pdf [Accessed September 28, 2019].

Uganda Bureau of Statistics (UBOS), 2011. *Uganda Demographic Health Survey*, Kampala. Available at: https://dhsprogram.com/pubs/pdf/FR264/FR264.pdf [Accessed September 28, 2019].

Uganda Bureau of Statistics (UBOS), 2006. *Uganda Demographic Health Survey*, Kampala. Available at: http://www.dhsprogram.com/pubs/pdf/FR194/FR194.pdf [Accessed September 28, 2019].

Umlauf, R., 2017. *Mobile Labore Zur Diagnose und Organisation von Malaria in Uganda*, Bielefeld: transcript.

United Nations (UN), 2015. *The Millennium Development Goals Report 2015*, New York. Available at: http://www.un.org/millenniumgoals/2015_MDG_Report/pdf/MDG 2015 rev (July 1).pdf [Accessed September 28, 2019].

United Nations (UN), 2015a. *Transforming our World: The 2030 Agenda for Sustainable Development A/RES/70/1*, Available at: https://sustainabledevelopment.un.org/content/documents/21252030 Agenda for Sustainable Development web.pdf [Accessed September 28, 2019].

United Nations (UN), 2011. *NCDs and MDGs – Success in Synergy*. Political declaration of the High-level Meeting of the General Assembly on the Prevention and Control of Non-Communicable Diseases, New York, 19-20 September 2011. Available at: http://www.who.int/nmh/events/un_ncd_summit2011/ncd_mdg.pdf?ua=1 [Accessed September 28, 2019].

United Nations (UN), 2007. *Africa and the Millennium Development Goals*, Available at: https://www.un.org/millenniumgoals/pdf/mdg2007.pdf [Accessed September 28, 2019].

United Nations (UN), 2000. *UN Millennium Declaration, 8th of September 2000*, New York. Available at: http://www.un.org/millennium/declaration/ares552e.htm [Accessed September 28, 2018].

van Crevel, R., van de Vijver, S. & Moore, D.A.J., 2017. The global diabetes epidemic: what does it mean for infectious diseases in tropical countries? *The Lancet Diabetes & Endocrinology*, 5(6), pp. 457–468. Available at: http://linkinghub.elsevier.com/retrieve/pii/S221385871630081X [Accessed September 28, 2019].

von Schnitzler, A., 2013. Traveling technologies: Infrastructure, ethical regimes, and the materiality of politics in South Africa. *Cultural Anthropology*, 28(4), pp. 670–693.

Warren, N. & Manderson, L., 2016. Credibility and the Inexplicable: Parkinson's Disease and Assumed Diagnosis in Contemporary Australia. In C. M. Smith-Morris, ed. *Diagnostic Controversy. Cultural Perspectives on Competing Knowledge in Healthcare*. New York/ London: Routledge, pp. 127–146.

Weaver, L.J. & Mendenhall, E., 2014. Applying syndemics and chronicity: interpretations from studies of poverty, depression, and diabetes. *Medical anthropology*, 33(2), pp. 92–108. Available at: http://www.ncbi.nlm.nih.gov/pubmed/24512380 [Accessed September 28, 2019].

Wendland, C.L., 2012. Moral maps and medical imaginaries: clinical tourism at Malawi's College of Medicine. *American anthropologist*, 114(1), pp. 108–22.

Wendland, C.L., 2010. *A heart for the work: journeys through an African medical school*, Chicago: University of Chicago Press.

Whyte, S. et al., 2015. The visibility of non-communicable diseases in Northern Uganda. *African Health Sciences*, 15(1), p. 82–89. Available at: http://www.ncbi.nlm.nih.gov/pubmed/25834534 [Accessed September 28, 2019].

Whyte, S., 2014a. Timeliness and chronic medication: knowledge about hypertension and diabetes in Uganda. *Working Papers of the Priority Programme 1448 of the German Research Foundation*, (7). Available at: https://lost-research-group.org/wp-content/uploads/2017/05/SPP1448_WP7_Susan_R_Whyte.pdf [Accessed September 28, 2019].

Whyte, S., 2014b. The Publics of the New Public Health. Life Conditions and "Lifestyle Diseases" in Uganda. In R. J. Prince & R. Marsland, eds. *Making and Unmaking Public Health in Africa*. Athens/ Ohio: Ohio University Press, pp. 187–207.

Whyte, S. et al., 2013. Therapeutic Clientship. Belonging in Uganda's Projectified Landscape of AIDS Care. In J. G. Biehl & A. Petryna, eds. *When People Come First*. Princeton, Oxford: Princeton University Press, pp. 140–165.

Whyte, S., 2012. Chronicity and control: framing "noncommunicable diseases" in Africa. *Anthropology & Medicine*, 19(1), pp. 63–74.

Will, C. & Moreira, T., 2010. *Medical proofs, social experiments clinical trials in shifting contexts* C. Will & T. Moreira, eds., Farnham and Burlington: Ashgate Publishing.

Witzel, A. & Reiter, H., 2012. *The problem-centred interview: principles and practice*, Thousand Oaks: SAGE Publications.

World Health Organization (WHO), 2017a. *Diabetes*, Geneva. Available at: http://www.who.int/mediacentre/factsheets/fs312/en/ [Accessed September 28, 2019].

World Health Organization (WHO), 2017b. *Noncommunicable diseases. Fact sheet*, Geneva. Available at: http://www.who.int/mediacentre/factsheets/fs355/en/ [Accessed September 28, 2019].

World Health Organization (WHO), 2017c. Knowledge translation. Available at: http://www.who.int/ageing/projects/knowledge_translation/en/ [Accessed September 29, 2019].

World Health Organization (WHO), 2016a. Global Report on Diabetes, p.88. Available at: http://apps.who.int/iris/bitstream/10665/204871/1/9789241565257_eng.pdf [Accessed September 28, 2019].

World Health Organization (WHO), 2016b. Integrated community case management of malaria. Available at: http://www.who.int/malaria/areas/community_case_management/overview/en/ [Accessed September 28, 2019].

World Health Organization (WHO), 2015. Knowledge translation framework for ageing and health. *WHO*. Available at: http://www.who.int/ageing/publications/knowledge_translation/en/ [Accessed September 28, 2019].

World Health Organization (WHO), 2011. *Accelerating the MDGs by addressing NCDs*, Available at: http://www.who.int/nmh/events/2010/discussion_paper_20100920.pdf [Accessed September 28, 2019].

World Health Organization (WHO), 2010. Package of essential noncommunicable disease interventions for primary health care in low-resource settings. *Geneva: World Health Organization*, p. 66.

World Health Organization (WHO), 2003. *STEPS: A framework for surveillance*, Geneva. Available at: http://www.who.int/ncd_surveillance/en/steps_framework_dec03.pdf [Accessed September 28, 2019].

World Health Organization (WHO), 1998a. *World Health Organization Organisation mondiale de la Santé. The world health report 1998, Life in the 21st century: a vision for all*, Available at: http://apps.who.int/gb/archive/pdf_files/WHA51/ea3.pdf [Accessed September 28, 2019].

World Health Organization (WHO), 1998b. *The World Health Report 1998 Life in the 21st century A vision for all*, Geneva. Available at: http://www.who.int/whr/1998/en/whr98_en.pdf?ua=1 [Accessed September 28, 2019].

World Health Organization (WHO), 1989. *WHA42.36 Prevention and Control of diabetes mellitus*, Geneva. Available at: http://www.who.int/diabetes/publications/en/wha_resol42.36.pdf [Accessed September 28, 2019].

World Health Organization (WHO) and International Diabetes Federation (IDF), 2006. *Definition and Diagnosis of Diabetes Mellitus and Intermediate Hyperglycemia*, Geneva. Available at: http://www.who.int/diabetes/publications/Definition%20and%20diagnosis%20of%20diabetes_new.pdf [Accessed September 28, 2019].

Yanow, D., 2004. Translating Local Knowledge at Organizational Peripheries. *British Journal of Management*, 15(S1), pp. 9–25. Available at: http://doi.wiley.com/10.1111/j.1467-8551.2004.t01-1-00403.x [Accessed September 28, 2019].

Young, A., 1981. When rational men fall sick: an inquiry into some assumptions made by medical anthropologists. *Culture, medicine and psychiatry*, 5(4), pp. 317–335.

Zimmet, P., Williams, J. & de Courten, M., 2002. Diabetes and classification of diabetes mellitus. In J. A. H. Wass & S. M. Shalet, eds. *Oxford Textbook of Endocrinology and Diabetes*. Oxford: Oxford University Press, pp. 1635–164.

GPSR Authorized Representative: Easy Access System Europe, Mustamäe tee 50, 10621 Tallinn, Estonia, gpsr.requests@easproject.com

www.ingramcontent.com/pod-product-compliance
Lightning Source LLC
Chambersburg PA
CBHW051538020426
42333CB00016B/1988